THE
PATH
OF THE
Mindful
TEACHER

How to choose calm over
chaos and serenity over stress,
one step at a time

DANIELLE A. NUHFER

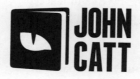

First published 2021

by John Catt Educational Ltd

15 Riduna Park, Station Road,
Melton, Woodbridge IP12 1QT
UK
Tel: +44 (0) 1394 389850

4500 140th Ave North,
Suite 101, Clearwater,
FL 33762-3848
US
Tel: +1 561 448 1987

Email: enquiries@johncatt.com
Website: www.johncatt.com

ISBN: 978 1 913622 61 9

Set and designed by John Catt Educational Limited

Endorsements

"*The Path of the Mindful Teacher* provides teachers with a roadmap for discerning what is in their control and what may be best to let go in order to increase serenity and calm both in the classroom and beyond. Creating boundaries through focusing on the vital few is sure to bring a more balanced quality to all parts of life, leading to a more satisfying teaching career."

Greg McKeown, author of *Essentialism: the disciplined pursuit of less*

"Speaks to the real challenges that teachers face, and actually provides ways to solve what they can control. Should be required reading for every first-year teacher, given to them by their principal, so they know what a healthy relationship with their work is. More than ever we need amazing teachers entering (and staying) in the profession. This book will help great teachers stay in the profession."

Jethro Jones, educator, author of *SchoolX*, and host of the *Transformative Principal* podcast

"Learning how to achieve mindfulness in education can seem daunting, but the path laid out in this book makes it an achievable goal for any teacher who knows that in order to grow through their burnout, they must do things they've never done. *The Path of the Mindful Teacher* is a wonderful reminder that living with intention starts with paying attention. With Danielle as your guide, you will have the opportunity to explore ways to pay more attention to your energy, choices, outlook, and influence, and how your focus on these things will truly help you go from stress to serenity and chaos to calm."

Amber Harper, author of *Hacking Teacher Burnout* and host of the *Burned-In Teacher* podcast

"Danielle writes a beautiful manifest about walking the Path of the Mindful Teacher – it is a must-read for current and preservice teachers alike. The way Danielle writes is conversational and informative, sharing tangible tips to help us all live a more mindful life as educators."

Dr. Samantha Fecich, host of the *EduMagic Future Teacher* podcast; author of *EduMagic: a guide for preservice teachers* and co-author of *EduMagic Shine On: a guide for new teachers*

"Almost every educator I have met nods and smiles knowingly while they agree that mindfulness is a good thing. But how many would couple mindfulness and teaching with the Serenity Prayer? Who would think there could be Four Noble Truths of Teaching? These ideas, along with practical practices illustrated with authentic stories from the classroom, are from teacher Danielle A. Nuhfer's new book *The Path of the Mindful Teacher*. She gives teachers ways to deal with the infinite number of stressful competing external demands: from developing a community of positive educators to offering a compendium of internal mindfulness practices from luminaries in the field. Not to mention the valuable practical, helpful habits that can used during 'one of those days' (or semesters, or years). You know the ones I mean. For some of us, using the ideas and practices in her book could be the difference between following a path leading to burnout or following the Path of the Mindful Teacher to thriving in the profession we love."

Kirke Olson, Psy.D, author of *The Invisible Classroom: relationships, neuroscience, and mindfulness in school*. www.thepositivitycompany.com

"In *The Path of the Mindful Teacher*, Danielle leads us on an alternative journey from our current path of chaos and stress to one of calm and serenity. Danielle gently nurtures teachers to be open to a more mindful existence and provides ways to do this in an inviting way. The book also covers many of my favourite topics, such as strengths, flow, and self-compassion. As a teacher who struggled with never-ending marking, unrealistic workloads, stress, and exhaustion, mindfulness has helped me to be a better teacher, a more mindful listener, and more importantly to respond to students instead of reacting. As Zen master Thich Nhat Hanh profoundly states, happy teachers change the world."

Patrice Palmer, M.Ed., M.A., author of *The Teacher Self-Care Manual*

"In a time where education is more important than ever, Danielle illuminates a mindful path of effective and compassionate education to benefit both students and their teachers. Highly recommended!"

Sean W. Murphy, Zen teacher, National Endowment for the Arts fellow in creative writing, and author of *One Bird, One Stone: 108 contemporary Zen stories* and three novels. www.murphyzen.com

"Have you found yourself wondering if teaching is no longer for you? Do you feel as if there is an endless and overwhelming amount that you must do as a teacher, to the point where there is no time left for you? Danielle joins you in having those experiences and will show you, through the Four Noble Truths of Teaching, how to get out of the tunnel and into the light. This remarkable, readable book will invigorate you, recharge you, and bring smiles to your face when you are in school. You will be the teacher you know you can be. While you will find this book to be a daily gift, the greatest gift will be how you see your students respond to the renewed you!"

Maurice J. Elias, Ph.D., professor of psychology at Rutgers University, director of the Social-Emotional and Character Development Lab, and co-author of *Nurturing Students' Character: everyday teaching activities for social-emotional learning*

Contents

Thank you to my students, who unknowingly encouraged me to discover this path and uncover the teacher and person who was waiting to be found.

No one saves us but ourselves.
No one can and no one may.
We ourselves must walk the path.
Buddha

As in all things,
simply begin again.

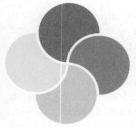

Introduction:
What is the Path of the
Mindful Teacher?

A journey of a thousand miles begins with a single step – Lao Tzu

Have you ever woken up one morning and not known how you got where you are? Not in a college party kind of way, but in a much bigger way. You don't recognize yourself any more. You aren't the person you aspired to be. You don't want to get out of bed because the world is running you in circles. You aren't sure who's calling the shots, but it certainly isn't you.

It couldn't be you. Could it?

How could you have *chosen* to pile up one responsibility after another, without ever considering that you might need a change of direction or a repair in your relationship with teaching?

How could you have *chosen* to add more tasks to your overflowing list of teacher to-dos, or chosen to take on another fundraiser in addition to all the grading sitting on your desk?

How could you have *chosen* to bring home worry after worry about other people's children, while your child sits at the table telling you about their day and you have to dig deep simply to try to be present with them?

You wouldn't have chosen this lather-rinse-repeat cycle of daily obligation, would you? And if you did, why? How did it get this far out of hand?

I want to share this news with you: you more than likely *did* choose the path you're currently on, but not because you enjoy the stress. You don't harbor deep-seated resentment against yourself. This wasn't a way to get back at yourself for a mistake. You didn't accrue lousy karma in a previous life.

No, you more than likely chose this path, like I did, because you care. You're passionate about what you do. You love working with children. You might have felt the drive, desire, and commitment to become a teacher from a young age. You chose this path because, at first, it felt good to say yes. It felt good to be the one to take care of everything. It felt manageable to add one more thing to the list. Someone had to do it, and you wanted to help your students more than anything.

As Lao Tzu writes, a journey begins with a single step. You kept walking and working toward that elusive payoff, conclusion, or gold star, but the path never ended. Perpetually, year after year, you kept walking toward a finish line that doesn't exist. Working harder only added to the stress and chaos. But, just as that journey began with a single step, you have another opportunity to step in a different direction and move toward serenity and calm. You can choose to walk the Path of the Mindful Teacher.

You may have been part of the problem, but you are also the solution. That's the secret I want to share: you can *choose* a different path. Instead of allowing stress to permeate your days, you can, believe it or not, choose serenity. Instead of allowing chaos to run you ragged, you can choose to create calm for yourself and your students.

I know because I've been through this myself. And guess what? Making different choices is not going to make you a less effective teacher. It's not going to encourage your students to feel like they're getting away with something. Choosing a different path – one that supports your life and those who depend on you – can even make you *more* effective. Your students may feel more seen and heard and cared for, and you may see their discipline problems in a new light.

Choosing the path of serenity over stress, and calm over chaos, won't cure all the woes of your school or your profession. But you will see in this book how you have a choice to do things differently, by walking the Path of the Mindful Teacher.

If you want some relief from the stress you're feeling, keep reading. This is a path I've traveled myself and I continue to walk it every day. I'm happy to be your guide.

Our stress is contagious

If you're still reading, congratulations! It's great that you've decided to choose a different path.

First, it's essential to get one simple fact out of the way: your stress is contagious. Of course, not all stress is bad – bursts of tension are great for achieving goals and staying accountable. But I'm referring to the pervasive stress that you feel day in, day out. It's toxic and it can spread.

If we carry toxic stress into our classrooms day after day, we infect our students, regardless of whether we're teaching them in a classroom or virtually. And before you say it, yes, I know: they also infect us with their stress. But we can't control that – we can only manage ourselves. We can fortify ourselves, building our resistance and resilience, and that's the Path of the Mindful Teacher. It's a practice we can use to counter the stress and overwhelm of being a teacher today.

Much of our job involves navigating students' social and emotional health, but we're asked to do this with little or no training in the field. If we want to continue this work we have a calling to do, we need to figure out how to take care of ourselves in our current reality.

I don't want to catalog all that's wrong with the US education system. That is well beyond the scope of this book. But I posit that if we learn how to choose calm over chaos and serenity over stress, we will alter our individual experiences, and potentially these differences will begin to change the system. When we are operating from a healthy, balanced foundation, we will demand what we need or create it somewhere else. Before we upend the entire system, however, we need to take the steps along the path and walk it, one teacher at a time. That's what this book is for.

Lest you start feeling ill at the thought of stress being contagious, here's a bright spot: our positive emotions are also contagious. This is good news. When we learn to choose serenity over stress, we can pass on our positive emotions to our students.

Of course, you can't fix each student. As much as we wish we had a magic wand to wave away all their problems and keep them all safe, we don't. What you *can* do is show up for your students every day, and be one of perhaps few adults in their lives to demonstrate how to be present and alert, develop a positive outlook, and implement healthy boundaries.

You can be the change you want to see in your world. You can be the change for your students. You can show them there is an alternative to being stressed out, running on autopilot, reacting to situations instead of responding. You can choose differently. So, let's get started!

What do you mean I have a choice?

To explain what I mean by choice, I've created the Four Noble Truths of Teaching. This phrasing is rooted in the Buddhist tradition – I borrowed the language because it works. This is, of course, a secular book and you don't need to become a Buddhist to travel down this path. Even the Buddha meant his Four Noble Truths to be for laypeople everywhere, not just practicing Buddhists. So, the Four Noble Truths of Teaching are meant for teachers everywhere to apply to their teaching lives.

The Buddha promised enlightenment to anyone who followed his Four Noble Truths. Although I'm not the Buddha, and I can't promise you enlightenment, I *can* promise you that by accepting the Four Noble Truths of Teaching, you will become empowered. And that could lead you down the path of enlightenment – at least as a classroom teacher.

I like to think of the Four Noble Truths of Teaching, presented on the opposite page, as a flow chart leading us from stress to serenity and chaos to calm…

The Four Noble Truths of Teaching

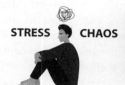
STRESS · CHAOS

First Noble Truth
The teaching life is difficult, full of stress and demands on our time and attention.

Second Noble Truth
Much of our stress comes from not knowing how to manage the external factors, often beyond our control, that impact our classrooms.

Third Noble Truth
There is a way to lessen the stress and demands, and to live a more balanced teaching life.

Fourth Noble Truth
The way to achieve serenity and calm is to make teaching less about what we can't control and more about what we can. To thrive, we must be mindful of our responses to external factors and nurturing to our internal lives.

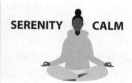
SERENITY · CALM

The First Noble Truth of Teaching

The teaching life is difficult, full of stress and demands on our time and attention.

Well, I think we've all noticed this, so it might be an easy truth to accept. Teaching involves a ton of demands. There are demands on our time, energy, health, and wellbeing. We are continually asked to do more with less. We are continually expected to create perfect little standardized test-takers, when many of our students struggle to focus because of all the other things going on in their lives.

To put it mildly, teaching is full of demands. Sometimes these demands are unreasonable and unfair, but the reality is that they are there. If we want to stay in this profession (which is a question you can feel free to ask yourself – this is a judgment-free zone), we need to work with these demands in a way that supports our health and wellbeing.

So, the First Noble Truth of Teaching asks you to accept that this profession can be complicated, full of stress, and place many demands on your time and energy. That's it. Nothing more, nothing less. Can you accept that this truth is pretty spot on? If so, it's time to move on to the next truth.

The Second Noble Truth of Teaching

Much of our stress comes from not knowing how to manage the external factors, often beyond our control, that impact our classrooms.

We've established that our job is a difficult one, full of ever-present and sometimes ever-increasing demands on our time. A lot is expected of us and our students. These expectations – coupled with the countless other tasks we're asked to perform and the reality of how much "stuff" students bring to our classrooms every day – are a lot to deal with.

This leads us to the Second Noble Truth of Teaching: much of our stress comes from not knowing how to manage these external factors, which are often out of our control. We can't usually control school and district-level demands. We can't control what our students did or didn't eat for breakfast, what they saw on the internet, or what they heard their parents arguing about.

Put down the bat you keep beating yourself up with and take a deep breath. With this truth, I'm asking you to take a big step – one that may feel a little uncomfortable or difficult. You may not even want to take it, but I'm asking you to "fake it until you make it."

Can you accept that external factors are the cause of a lot of your stress *and* that these things are out of your control? It's essential to be truthful about their being beyond your control. Of course, teachers are on the front lines demanding less testing, more funding, and advocating for children's wellbeing. We show up at fundraising events, make cookies for the bake sale, and donate money to these causes. I'm not suggesting you stop doing these things or let go of your passion. Absolutely not. What I want you to try to see is that these things we're fighting to change will change in their own time, on their own terms, pushed and prodded along by teachers like you and me. But, of course, that doesn't change the fact that these external factors are showing up *now*, day after day, and impacting your classroom. The powerlessness we feel around these issues can crank up our stress.

I ask you to open your heart and mind, and take an honest appraisal of your classroom. Can you accept that much of the stress that permeates your classroom results from factors beyond your control? If you can't say that *much* of it is out of your control, can you say that at least *some* of it is?

If you can answer yes to either of those questions, it's time to move on to the next truth.

The Third Noble Truth of Teaching

There is a way to lessen the stress and demands, and to live a more balanced teaching life.

In the Second Noble Truth, I asked you to accept your powerlessness over the external factors that impact your classroom day after day. I knew it would be hard for you to accept that. But I also knew what the next truth was going to be, and it takes us into the upswing of empowerment. There is a solution.

I don't know how many teachers have said to me that they just want to "do their job." This means something a little different depending on who and what they teach, but what each educator is essentially saying is that they want to work with kids. They want to improve the lives of their students; to help them learn something and be a more productive member of society. Quite simply, educators want to do the job they were trained to do and leave all the other stuff at the door.

The Third Noble Truth promises that you will have less stress, fewer demands, and be able to live a more balanced teaching life. That's a pretty hefty promise, but it will come to fruition if you commit and keep reading.

In your heart, you may not believe me. You may be reasonably skeptical. You may fear that I'm going to ask you to turn off your caring nature to avoid the realities of the stress in your classroom. Fear not. I won't be asking anything like that. You just need to have a little hope that a more balanced teaching life is possible. You also need to *want* what these truths are offering. The Buddha offered enlightenment. The Four Noble Truths of Teaching are offering a more balanced, less stressed teaching life, and that might be pretty close to a feeling of enlightenment. It may feel pretty enlightening to come to work every day, do your job, and teach your students, but not bear the burdens and not be bogged down by all the stuff beyond your control.

Instead of enlightenment, I use the words "serenity" and "calm." By working through these truths and the rest of this book, you may at least find a sense of serenity and calm in your classroom that perhaps you have been unable to access before. So, are you ready to move on to the solution?

The Fourth Noble Truth of Teaching

The way to achieve serenity and calm is to make teaching less about what we can't control and more about what we can. To thrive, we must be mindful of our responses to external factors and nurturing to our internal lives.

There it is. Ta-da! The Fourth Noble Truth of Teaching promises that we will thrive if we become mindful about how we respond to those pesky external factors, while learning to nurture our inner lives. By keeping the focus on ourselves, we will begin to be able to choose serenity over stress in our classrooms. This truth may feel empowering, because the solution lies within us. But it may also feel daunting.

There's a famous quote that's been attributed to everyone from Henry Ford to Tony Robbins and Jessie Potter: "If you want to keep getting what you're getting, keep doing what you're doing." If you want to get something different, you have to *do* something different. The empowering fact is that you can *choose* serenity over stress.

This choice is ultimately the Path of the Mindful Teacher. If you're ready to find out what that means, and to do something different so you can get something different, I invite you to keep turning these pages.

A note on the Serenity Prayer

In my desperate need to find something to help me move from chaos to calm, I've found inspiration from all corners of the world. Part of the reason I'm writing this book is to take all those bits of wisdom and show how they can influence our teaching practice, helping us get back to the basics of why we became teachers in the first place.

For example, the Serenity Prayer can be seen as a condensed version of the Four Noble Truths of Teaching. By committing it to memory and referring to it during times of stress, you may be able to find some space between the stimulus and your response. I offer this as a shortcut because I have found it useful, and because it has served as part of this book's inspiration.

Grant me the serenity to accept the things I cannot change,
courage to change the things I can,
and wisdom to know the difference.
– Reinhold Niebuhr

The Serenity Prayer asks us to be honest about what we can and can't change, and accept those things as they are. It suggests that we may be wise to know the difference. It indicates that by accepting those things we don't have control over (external factors) and being courageous enough to change the things we do have control over (ourselves), we may find some serenity.

This is simple in theory, and I'm sure you've heard this advice before, but it can be hard in practice. One of the main reasons it can be so difficult is that teaching is a caring profession. We often feel like the people who need to be cared for first and foremost are our students. I'm going to ask you to shelve that assumption for the duration of this book.

As we move forward, I offer the Serenity Prayer as a means of remembering that we can *choose* serenity over stress, by letting go of what we can't control and moving into action on the things we can. That is what the rest of this book offers you. It will help you cultivate the wisdom to discern the things you cannot change from the things you can.

In the chapters that follow, I will suggest mindfulness practices for you to try. I'll give you resources to refer to at the end of each chapter, and additional reading recommendations that may provide the data you desire. There may be some numbers within these pages, but that's not what this book is about. My goal is to offer actionable items to help you choose calm over chaos and serenity over stress. I have read the research and this book will provide you with a way to put all the research into action.

What is the Path of the Mindful Teacher?

I'm a teacher, and I've worked with thousands of fellow teachers. Their stories and struggles are the reason I've developed the Path of the Mindful Teacher. But let me begin by describing the path of the not-mindful teacher – see if you can relate to it.

Not-mindful teachers believe that doing everything for everybody else makes them good at their jobs. Sacrificing themselves, their sanity, their health, and their wellbeing is seen as a badge of honor that helps them do the job of caring for other people's children.

I went down this road. I was the person who took on too many things. I filled my calendar because that made me feel like I was helping people – making a difference. I knew these responsibilities wouldn't make me rich or famous. I was a teacher, for goodness sake – no one goes into teaching for the money. But what I didn't realize was that my self-worth had become directly proportional to how many responsibilities I shouldered. I didn't recognize it at the time, but my ego was saying yes when everything in my body was telling me no.

I remember talking to my husband the night before I was to decide about taking on the responsibility of being the yearbook advisor. This was not something I had ever aspired to do. Back in high school, for my class yearbook, I was nominated "most involved" in the Senior "bests." That was the first indication that I had an aversion to saying no, or an overextended ego. Now I think about it, that simply meant that I did many things, but probably none of them well. My nose was in everything, yet I couldn't commit.

But now, I was talking to my husband about taking on this extraordinary commitment on top of all the other responsibilities of teaching. I remember our conversation vividly. We talked about the pros and cons. Everything pointed in the direction of doing it: I would get paid extra, work with students in a creative way, and have an end product that would represent why I was doing what I was doing in my classroom each day. On paper, it looked like a done deal, except for the bowling ball in the pit of my stomach and the screaming voice in my head urging me to abort the mission. But I shoved those feelings to one side and accepted the role.

My first year in charge was overwhelming, to say the least. I became yearbook advisor mid-production. I didn't know the students, the technology, or the process. I managed, but it was relentless and tiring. Thank goodness the room was full of capable and conscientious students who really knew what they were doing.

The next year was another year of learning. Another year of doing. Another year of deadlines and mounting stress. Honestly, it wasn't just the yearbook project – it was everything else I hadn't let go of when I decided to take on this new responsibility. And, even more honestly, this responsibility didn't really work with my strengths. I'm an introvert. I love being in a classroom with my students, talking about literature and working with them on writing. I'm not one who likes to market, promote, or cheerlead. I'm not one who is in the spotlight fielding phone calls from parents about senior ads or payment options. I like to keep to myself and work with my students. It wasn't a good match and my stress level was letting me know that.

Taking on this ill-fitting responsibility without giving up any of my other duties eventually brought me to my knees. It was August, my third year as yearbook advisor, and back-to-school anticipation was in the air. But with that came the dreadful realization of all the work, responsibilities, and commitments I had shouldered as a result of saying yes. I usually welcomed the hustle and bustle of making calendars and copies. There's a natural order to the cycle of teaching, and it usually felt good and stable and right. But not this year.

I started to panic. I wanted to escape, but the clock was ticking. I knew the students' demands and all the other responsibilities would soon come rushing back, whether I was ready or not.

I contemplated quitting. I considered not showing up. I searched for other jobs. I melted down at a friend's house, crying hysterically that I couldn't go back. My nervous system felt overloaded just *thinking* about the deadlines, the responsibilities, the needs that I was expected to meet, the stark reality that I couldn't even meet my own needs – and they would surely be last on the list.

It was clear something needed to change, but what exactly was going on? Was it me? Was it the job? Was it something else entirely? Ultimately, I didn't quit my job, but I didn't continue on the same path. I couldn't have continued on the same path if I wanted to live a life beyond burnout.

Everyone is different in what they need. I stood on a precipice: I could either walk away from teaching entirely, or choose to do something different. I opted to take an educational sabbatical and I discovered mindfulness in education. At first, I thought it was about getting this effective practice to students, but instead it became about creating a personal practice *first* and then teaching the skills to students. I was consistently reminded about putting the oxygen mask on myself first.

During this time, I started to learn about the prevalence of teacher burnout. I started to learn about how stress is contagious. I started to realize that there were solutions to the intense anxiety I had experienced, and one possible solution was a regular mindfulness practice. I studied more and more, and eventually, when I returned to my teaching job, I began sharing these findings with fellow teachers. I went on to start Teaching Well, which helps teachers prioritize and nourish themselves to increase wellbeing and decrease burnout.

I had been the garden-variety not-mindful teacher who believed this was just how teaching was and this was how I would always feel. Well, here's a mantra that I want you to repeat when you feel like there isn't enough of you to go around:

This is common, but not normal.

Yes, it is so common – too common – for teachers to slide, year after year, deeper and deeper into a fog of stress and overwhelm. But if this phenomenon continues to be normalized, we will continue to accept it as part of the profession.

This weight of stress and the potential burnout do not serve us professionally or personally. They do not serve our students' needs. They do not serve the larger stakeholders in our communities and nation.

I'm sure we all have a story of overload and overwhelm. Every teacher's story is different, but the outcomes are relatively similar. When the pressures mount, when the stress builds, we have only a few options:

1. Quit teaching entirely.
2. Hunker down and do the job at the expense of our wellbeing.
3. Change something.

None of these options seem particularly easy, obvious, or appealing. Option 2 is the one many of us choose. We are hard workers. We don't want to complain about the expectations, the behavior issues, the mounting workload with diminishing resources. But the problem with "hunkering down" is that everything else suffers, and you may resort to Option 1 because you're at your wit's end.

If you've spent a long time depleting your wellbeing, and piling on the guilt and shame to such a degree that you can't do the job you're expected to do, you may choose Option 1 because you don't feel there's another way. What could change enough to help you get out of bed in the morning and look forward to your job? After months and years of plugging away, it may be hard to see that change is a possibility. But Option 3 is available to us all.

Perhaps you're not at the point of quitting, or even suffering the effects of years of taking on too much for too little. But maybe you're on your way. Statistically, it's likely that you're stressed: in a recent study, 93% of elementary school teachers reported high stress levels and burnout symptoms.[1] At the very least, if you're reading this book, you probably feel compelled to bring more serenity to your classroom and tackle the stress that often disguises itself as "jobs that need doing."

Regardless of where you are on the stress scale, if you're even remotely feeling some dread and overwhelm, I ask you to choose Option 3. Your job doesn't have to be the way it is right now. You don't need to feel the way you're feeling right now. You do have the ability to make changes that can bring serenity to your day. It may not happen immediately. It may not be a complete cure-all, but I promise that if you can shift your thinking, you may be surprised at how good you end up feeling.

---

1. Herman, K.C., Hickmon-Rosa, J., & Reinke, W.M. (2017) Empirically derived profiles of teacher stress, burnout, self-efficacy, and coping and associated student outcomes. *Journal of Positive Behavior Interventions*, 20(2), 90-100

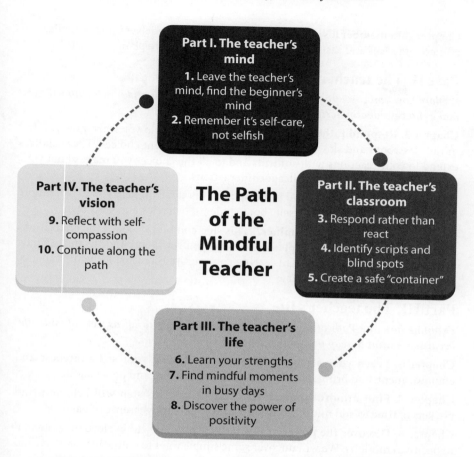

So, there it is. There is the Path of the Mindful Teacher. There are four parts to this journey, and each part contains several steps, each of which will be explored in its own chapter.

Part I. The teacher's mind

Set up a mindfulness practice and commit to self-care, because a healthy teacher has a healthy mind.

Chapter 1. Leave the teacher's mind, find the beginner's mind. This step asks you to become a student again and learn some new tools. We will learn about mindfulness and what that means, and what mindfulness practice looks like in our personal and professional lives.

Chapter 2. Remember it's self-care, not selfish. This step delves into the application of these practices and assists you in creating your self-care plan.

Part II. The teacher's classroom

Explore how you can apply mindfulness to your classroom and how it can help you make choices, identify scripts, and build relationships.

Chapter 3. Respond rather than react. This step will help you learn how you feel in the classroom and slow down enough to make different choices. These choices extend to your reactions with students and to all the choices you make about your duties, responsibilities, and colleague interactions.

Chapter 4. Identify scripts and blind spots. This step will help you explore more deeply the stories you tell yourself about students' behavior and your own.

Chapter 5. Create a safe "container." This step combines a lot of the realizations made in the previous two chapters, and helps you work on building an authentic and meaningful community. This caring community is created for your students, but you will also be a beneficiary.

Part III. The teacher's life

Examine how the Path of the Mindful Teacher extends to all aspects of your life, because we want to reap these benefits in school and beyond.

Chapter 6. Learn your strengths. This step will build your self-awareness and empowerment, and bring more ease to your professional and personal life.

Chapter 7. Find mindful moments in busy days. This step will help you find pockets of time to add mindfulness to your days, creating a sense of balance.

Chapter 8. Discover the power of positivity. This step will explore the potential of positive emotions. We will uncover some simple ways to cultivate positivity, and see how this practice can help to transform wellbeing from the inside out.

Part IV. The teacher's vision

Recognize your role in continuing this work in your classroom and perhaps beyond, into the wider world of education.

Chapter 9. Reflect with self-compassion. This step considers the importance of reflective teaching practices, and asks you to bring self-compassion to those practices to ensure honesty in your reflections.

Chapter 10. Continue along the path. This step takes a look back at the work we've done and charts a course for the future. You now have a solution to the stress that permeates your classroom. What will you choose to do to move forward?

Let's make this clear: when it comes to walking the Path of the Mindful Teacher, the joy is in the journey. We're never really done. You will never "arrive." Instead, you will travel along the path and return to the beginning, where you will be different. Should you choose to walk the path again, you will experience it differently.

It may be helpful to read the whole book, then revisit the activities at the end of each chapter once you know where you're being taken. Or it may be beneficial to do some of the activities as you read. I invite you to work with this book in the way that calls to you. There is no "right" way.

This book is written as a gift to all teachers, current and future. The words are an offering of my experience, strength, and hope. May you take the work into your world as you see fit for your specific circumstance.

Questions to ponder on the path

- How is your stress contagious (as well as your other emotions)?
- What potential hindrances cause stress and chaos in your classroom?
- What potential solutions can help you find serenity and calm in your classroom?
- What is the Path of the Mindful Teacher, and what immediate steps can you take to move forward?

Step into action

- Create one classroom goal inspired by what you've learned about the Four Noble Truths of Teaching.
- Create one classroom or personal goal you would like to work toward as you walk the Path of the Mindful Teacher.
- Write these down and keep them somewhere visible as you read the book.

Supplemental resources

Check out www.teachingwell.life/pathbook for more resources to accompany this chapter.

Part I.
The teacher's mind

Set up a mindfulness practice and commit to self-care, because a healthy teacher has a healthy mind

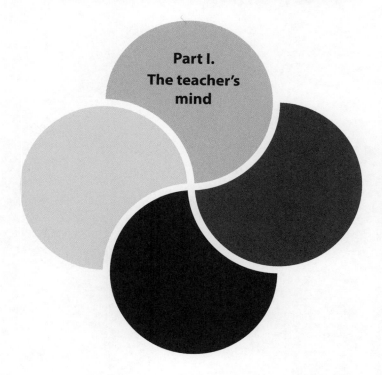

Part I.
The teacher's mind

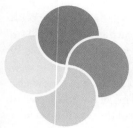

Chapter 1.
Leave the teacher's mind,
find the beginner's mind

In the beginner's mind there are many possibilities, but in the expert's there are few
– Shunryu Suzuki

Chapter objectives

You will be able to:

- Recognize the needs of your students and yourself.
- Understand what you have control over in your classroom, and how that can impact you and your students.
- Identify your beliefs about self-care and mindfulness, and determine what can be let go of and what can be held on to.

I started my semester of student teaching in the fall of 2001. When I state that, I always like to pose this question: in the US, what two key factors were at play during that time? People always remember the attacks on the Twin Towers on 9/11, but many forget this was also the year that the No Child Left Behind Act (NCLB) was passed, becoming law in 2002.

While 9/11 shook the country in a way none of us could have imagined, NCLB shook the public education system in a way it has still not fully recovered from. Over the previous four years, I had learned how to encourage student portfolio work and creativity, and how to use books to talk about social situations. With NCLB's mandate, all that kind of went out the window overnight. I didn't have much support where I was working because, of course, everyone else was trying to figure it out too.

I was fresh out of college, so I had a beginner's mind. I didn't know how else school was supposed to be, so I took what I knew and tried to make it work. I tried to play the NCLB game while figuring out ways to salvage some of those skills, because I knew they were the reason I had become a teacher. I saw possibilities to try new things and see what happened. I sometimes felt like I was going rogue, but, for the most part, I was able to ebb and flow with what was expected over the first few years.

This was not the experience of so many other, more experienced teachers. Many decided to retire because of all the changes. The transformation wasn't so jarring for me – *everything* had changed for me at that point in my career. I didn't know what would work and what wouldn't, because I lacked prior experience. At this moment, that was a blessing.

Full disclosure: I also identify NCLB as one reason why so many teachers who joined the profession during this time ended up leaving around year five (including me, and I'll get to that a little later). But having a beginner's mind during the first year or two of teaching saved me.

I'm going to ask you to apply this same concept to your current experience of teaching. Try to access your beginner's mind and allow yourself to consider the possibility that there is another path. Don't worry, you don't have to start entirely from scratch, but, for the duration of this book, can you let go of everything you think you know and try to walk this path with the beginner's mind? Nothing else has to change, but everything will change if you change.

This may not be comfortable or feel natural, because I'm asking you to become the student here. However, in some ways, it might be easier than you think, because we teachers are always learning, learning, learning. We remain consistently teachable as new and different initiatives cycle through.

Acknowledge where you are

Look at the current situation in your classroom and be honest. Is all of it working? Are you making progress? Hitting goals? Are you eating at your desk day after day, trying to make headway on all the different tasks? Is work spilling into other facets of your life? Or perhaps you're completely disengaged? Perhaps you've given up on the thought of things being different? Do you white-knuckle ride through your days and weeks, trying to tick off one more item so you can then relax, let go, breathe?

To begin to move from stress to serenity and chaos to calm, you need to acknowledge where you are. It's not about judging yourself. Do we judge our students for not knowing a concept? Well, maybe sometimes, but we also know that, as professionals, we need to move past the judgment and try to teach them.

Why do we think we should treat ourselves any differently than we treat our students? It takes time to learn and apply new concepts. Have you ever had to scrap a lesson because it landed wrong? You thought you had built the knowledge, but the kids didn't grasp it. As they say when constructing a house, if you don't build a strong foundation, the house will eventually crumble.

So, if we need to rebuild, we need to see things as they are, not as we wish them to be. This is a great place to refer to the Serenity Prayer for a little guidance: let's build some courage to change the things we can. Let's lean on our Fourth Noble Truth of Teaching: to thrive, we must be mindful of our responses to external factors and nurturing to our internal lives.

You don't have to be anxious or upset about not having it all figured out. You don't have to pretend that it's going well if it's not. Similarly, you don't have to pretend you have any real issues if things are feeling pretty good. Acknowledging where you are is not about shaming yourself if you feel like you're falling apart, or catastrophizing if this year was actually a pretty good one.

No matter what's happening in your classroom (pleasant and unpleasant), mindfulness will help you learn to respond rather than react. It's important to emphasize the fact that mindfulness is a *skill* you can *develop*. It's not something that you have or you don't – I can't stress this enough. That's why we think about this as a path: each step develops us more and more. With enough practice, you'll be able to walk the Path of the Mindful Teacher and see your classroom with new awareness. You'll interact with your students and yourself with more presence.

So, let's start practicing those skills!

It's time to get honest

Find a piece of paper and set a timer for the amount of time you have right now (maybe 10 minutes). On one side of the piece of paper, make two columns:

1. What are you already doing to support students?
2. What do your students need?

Write down everything you can think of and circle the ones you have direct control over. Now flip the paper over and make two more columns:

1. What are you already doing to support yourself? (If you can't think of anything, write down that you're reading this book and making this list!)

2. What do you need as an educator (physically, mentally, emotionally)?

Again, once you've made these lists, circle the things you have direct control over. Now you can see clearly what you're already doing to support your students and yourself. All hope is *not* lost. You can also see clearly which needs you have direct control over. You are *not* powerless.

Keep hold of that piece of paper. Perhaps use it as a bookmark or put it somewhere for easy reference as you read the book (and afterwards), because as we walk this path, we may get busy or distracted. Eventually we'll return to the start of the path, and we'll need to come back to being honest, clearing what we thought we knew, getting curious about what's going on, forgetting our teacher's mind, and bringing our beginner's mind to the fore. When in your life have you ever had to forget everything you thought you knew and try to be a learner again? The Path of the Mindful Teacher asks you to do that before you embark on learning the tools and developing the skills.

Now, find another piece of paper. It's time to get honest about your fears in letting go of what you believe to be true. Set a timer for the time you have and get honest about the following questions:

1. What are your feelings about letting go of your teacher's mind and finding your beginner's mind, when it comes to teaching and your classroom?

2. What are your fears?

3. What are you willing to let go of?

4. What do you think you'll have difficulty letting go of?

5. If you can access your beginner's mind, what do you want your classroom to look like when your first cycle of the path is completed? How do you want to feel?

Great! Now you have a sketch of how you feel in this moment and an honest appraisal of what you believe to be holding you back. You have a vision for where you want this journey to take you.

Ready for change

I want to acknowledge that this is hard work, especially when we've been in the teaching seat for so long. It may be challenging to let your guard down and trust that it's OK not to know. It's OK not to have it all figured out. It's OK not to be in the lead. It's OK to just be with what's happening right now. I've heard so many different teachers express their apprehension that mindfulness might not be the answer. But, after working through this book's exact activities, they can see the profound impact on their teaching, their connection with students, and how they relate to themselves. And I'll let you in on a secret: this skill will permeate all facets of your life. We'll look at mindfulness through a teaching lens, because I've witnessed the benefits it can have in a classroom setting, but it doesn't have to stop there. In fact, it won't stop there, even if you try to compartmentalize. You see, as you develop this skill, you will change your brain. This is something we'll explore further as we walk the path.

Before we embark on this journey, there's one more thing we need to address. We need to acknowledge our feelings and attitudes toward mindfulness and self-care. In some circles, these are buzzwords that have connotations of indulgence and luxury. They often conjure images of sitting cross-legged in a peaceful Zen garden.

I want you to write down how you *really* feel and what you *really* think about these concepts. Don't hold back. Let it rip. Again, we're starting where we are. Set a timer for the time you have and consider the following questions:

1. What do you think of when you hear the word "mindfulness"?
2. What do you think of when you hear the word "self-care"?
3. How do you feel when you think of learning about those ideas?
4. Challenge yourself: why do you think that way?
5. How will you let go of your perceptions (whatever they are) and access your beginner's mind?

It's important to note and be honest about these thoughts and feelings. But, remember, I'm asking you to pause those perceptions and embrace your beginner's mind when it comes to mindfulness and self-care.

Now you have a plan for how to start this journey. It reminds me of when my husband and I packed our backpacks for a camping trip. We got to the head of the trail and realized we had *way too much stuff*. We unloaded a lot of things from our backpacks into the car before we set off. Then we took the trip, got back to our car, and realized how much of the remaining stuff we wouldn't need the next time.

That's what this path is like. We've arrived at the beginning of our journey. To make it as successful as possible, we must unload some of the things we won't need as we walk the path. Otherwise, our bags will be too heavy.

Thank you for letting go of what you won't need on this journey. As you travel along the path, you'll probably realize that you brought along some other things that you don't need. Feel free to let them go on the way, or make a note to unload them for the next time. Now our bags are packed – with essentials only! – it's time to dive in and take the next step on the Path of the Mindful Teacher.

Questions to ponder on the path

- What is the current state of your classroom? What are your needs? What are your students' needs?
- What can you do to support the students you have? What can you do to support yourself?
- What beliefs can you let go of? What things are you no longer going to worry about?

Step into action

- Keep a copy of the Serenity Prayer somewhere visible, and check in about what is in your control and what's not.
- Display the lists you made in this chapter somewhere visible. Focus only on those things you can control.

Featured five-minute practice: Breath/Sound Awareness

- Set your timer for five minutes (or more).
- Begin focusing on your inhales and exhales.
- Try to identify where you feel your breath the most. This is your anchor, your home base.
- Spend some time trying to identify sounds inside and outside the room.
- Come back to your breath anchor until the time is up.

Supplemental resources

Check out www.teachingwell.life/pathbook for more resources to accompany this chapter.

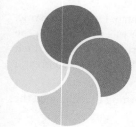

Chapter 2.
Remember it's self-care, not selfish

Two roads diverged in a wood, and I—
I took the one less traveled by,
And that has made all the difference – Robert Frost

Chapter objectives

You will be able to:

- Recognize what mindfulness is and is not.
- Practice adding mindful moments to daily and weekly schedules.
- Develop a self-care plan.

In 2012, I attended the Mindfulness and Education conference at the Omega Institute in Rhinebeck, New York. After hearing the inspirational speakers, meeting the fellow teachers, sharing stories, feeling the energy and the hope, I knew mindfulness was something I wanted to "do." I felt I had discovered the solution to so many of the problems in my classroom.

But as I sat in my seat on the last day, half-listening to the final speaker, I wasn't exactly the picture of mindfulness in action: I was nervously strategizing, scribbling notes, pausing, pondering. What could I cut to make time for mindfulness lessons for students? Which principal should I speak with to make sure this was added to all teachers' classrooms? Which teachers would want to hold group practices with me after school? Or before school? Perhaps I could drive to work and get there early?

My mind was racing. The pit of my stomach began to churn. I started to panic. This was how I felt every day – and this supposed antidote was now causing the same symptoms. It had not yet dawned on me that I was part of the problem. I felt nauseous. I could feel the dread settling in. But this mindfulness stuff is so great, I thought to myself. I can't just sit and do nothing.

At the end of that thought, I heard the speaker say something that changed the scope and trajectory of the next few years of my teaching.

Start with yourself first, because you can't transmit something you don't have.

We're talking about putting the oxygen mask on yourself first. You need to help yourself before you can help anybody else. This step on the Path of the Mindful Teacher is "remember it's self-care, not selfish." It's about letting go of the need to immediately introduce mindfulness to your students and first focus on putting your own practice in place. *Start with yourself first, because you can't transmit something you don't have.*

As I sat at the conference, I let the speaker's words sink in enough that I put down my pen and began to listen a little more. Then she said something that I tell all the teachers I work with. It was like the clouds had opened up and the sun was shining down upon me. I felt completely liberated.

You never even have to utter the word "mindfulness" to your students, but if you have your own personal practice, they will benefit because you are changing.

I hadn't been taught the idea of stress contagion at that point, but I trusted the speaker enough to believe what she was saying. I believed her for the sake of my sanity. I believed her because if I didn't, I was sure to carry on overloading myself and would do my students no good at all.

I let go of all my plans, for the moment, and gave myself permission to focus on developing these skills and tools for me, first. If I felt like doing something mindful in my classroom or talking about mindfulness to other teachers, I could, but this was a no-pressure zone. I gave myself a year to keep it about me. It was the first time I had been excited about something in my classroom that was purely for me, but that my students would benefit from.

If I'm honest, I wasn't sure that I completely believed a change would occur. Still, I decided to do something different. I decided to take the road less traveled, the one that encourages my self-care and wellbeing, in the hope that some of it would transmit to my students. Thank goodness I heard what the final speaker said. I paid enough attention to hear her words, and I decided to trust them.

In a short time, I diligently and wholeheartedly pieced together different books, resources, and practices, and I changed. My students' circumstances didn't change.

My school didn't get rid of standardized testing. I didn't become best friends with all my coworkers. But none of that mattered because, through the experience, I had changed. The way I showed up in my classroom had changed.

So, remember those words of wisdom from that sage speaker:

Start with yourself first, because you can't transmit something you don't have.

You never even have to utter the word "mindfulness" to your students, but if you have your own personal practice, they will benefit because you are changing.

I hope these words will help you choose calm over chaos and serenity over stress. This book asks you to begin to balance that tendency to always reach out, by instead reaching in. Eventually, you will be able to reach out when needed and reach in when you're off-balance. This is called equanimity, and we'll get there, but first we need to remember that it's self-care, not selfish.

Mindfulness basics

You may already know some things about mindfulness, or have a practice of your own, but it's good to be reminded to care for yourself first. We often forget that, despite our best intentions.

Let's review what we've already learned in this book:

- You can *choose* calm over chaos and serenity over stress.
- Much of our stress is caused by external factors. To thrive as educators, we must be mindful of our responses to those external factors and nurturing to our internal lives.
- The Path of the Mindful Teacher is the process of accepting our lack of control over those external factors and focusing on what we *can* control.
- To walk this path, we need to let go of our prior beliefs about self-care or mindfulness, returning to our beginner's mind to see if these concepts can work for us.

So, with these learnings in mind, let's take a look at what mindfulness is *not*. It's certainly a buzzword today – and a very misunderstood one. Mindfulness is not:

- Escaping from reality.
- Chanting.
- Doing yoga.
- Subscribing to a religion.
- Doing it "right."
- Changing your thoughts or feelings.

Are you ready for what it is?

Mindfulness is simply paying attention. That's it. *Mindfulness is being aware of what you're doing, when you're doing it, without judgment.*

I started this book by talking about the problem of teacher stress, because if I'd opened with that simple statement, you surely would have laughed that I'd written a whole book about paying attention. But although mindfulness isn't complicated, it's not easy either. Let's try it.

Get into a comfortable position and sit for 60 seconds. Just let yourself sit...

How was that? Did any thoughts bubble up? Were you surprised by how long or short 60 seconds felt? Did you notice anything about your breathing? What about your emotions? How did it feel to sit and do "nothing"?

Mindfulness is simple, but not always easy.

Everyone experiences mindfulness differently, and differently from day to day. This 60-second experience probably won't perfectly match other experiences that you have with it. As you practice, you'll build mindful muscles that will help you access serenity more readily. Later in the book, we'll look at how mindfulness can help you destress and decompress, and learn to respond rather than react in the classroom. Don't worry: there's science to back-up the experience.

Sitting still and focusing on something specific – like breathing, sound, or bodily sensations – is one kind of mindfulness practice. This is the kind of practice usually associated with mindfulness. But remember that mindfulness is simply paying attention to what you're doing, when you're doing it. And that means you can practice mindfulness anywhere, any time.

I'm going to describe four different types of mindfulness practice, and you can decide how you want to start. I suggest finding the path of least resistance – something you can implement quickly and without too much effort. Remember, you're just getting started, and we want to begin to feel some change from stress to serenity and chaos to calm as soon as possible.

Practice option #1: everyday activities

As we've already seen, you can apply mindfulness to any activity. Mindfulness is paying attention to what you're doing, when you're doing it, without judgment. So you can be mindful when you're washing the dishes, brushing your teeth, driving your car, going for a walk or run, or eating your meals.

Consider how often you do those activities mindlessly, distracting yourself with music, TV, phone, thoughts, or anything else that keeps you from fully being present with what you're doing. If you're like most humans on the planet, you spend much of your time completing tasks distractedly.

For example, have you ever driven from point A to point B, but not been able to recall much of the journey? That's downright scary, but most of us have done that at some point.

Have you ever sat down to watch a show with your favorite snack, and eaten the whole bag without realizing it?

Do you ever truly focus on what you're doing when you're putting the dishes away, brushing your teeth, folding your laundry?

I invite you to try to be mindful today of all the little tasks you perform. Which ones do you pay attention to? Which ones do you try to distract yourself during? Don't judge, just observe. Remember, we're experimenting.

After you've spent some time observing your patterns, try bringing full awareness to an activity or two during your day. Perhaps you could leave your phone at home when you go for a walk, or turn off the radio when you're folding laundry. Perhaps you could sit down for a meal, instead of eating in the car when you're running the kids around or grabbing a snack when you're between activities.

We're practicing with these small activities to get us ready for those moments that aren't mundane – those moments that can be stressful or chaotic. You know, those moments in your classroom!

Practice option #2: personal mindfulness practice

This practice is what you probably associate with mindfulness. We call it a "practice" because you're essentially exercising your brain when you sit and pay attention in a specific (mindful) way.

The main components of a personal mindfulness practice are **place, time, tool**:

1. The **place** is where you'll practice.
2. The **time** is when you'll show up to practice regularly.
3. The **tool** is what you'll use to guide or time you.

Find your place

You don't need a "perfect" place for this practice, just somewhere that's good enough. The places where I've chosen to practice mindfulness have changed and varied dramatically over the years. Depending on where I lived and whom I shared space with, I determined what was feasible. And guess what? You can always change when the circumstances change.

You might choose a favorite chair in a room; you might have a little space in your attic or a basement corner. I've seen people choose a space in their kitchen or a seat at their dining table. Depending on the time of day, you can repurpose any spot that's comfortable to you as the place where you can get into the habit of sitting for a few moments.

You may find that the best place is in bed before your feet hit the floor in the morning, or in your car before or after work. Your bathroom may be the only space you can find peace for a few moments. If that's the case, embrace it and know that you can change things up, if and when you're able to.

Find your time

By time, I mean the time of day when you'd like to practice. Your place may dictate your time, or the time you choose may dictate your place. Whichever comes first, make sure they work in harmony, and in a way that's practical for you and your current situation.

Some people identify as night owls or early birds. Some people like to take a few minutes before or after school. Some like to do their practice to wind down and fall asleep. Pick the time that will allow you to practice most easily. Some like to take it day by day; others create a rough routine. We're just beginning to walk this path, so we're keeping it simple. Choose a time, see how it goes, and modify as you need to.

Find your tool

Your tool is what you'll use to facilitate your mindfulness practice. You can do a silent practice by simply setting a timer on your phone. And if you prefer a silent practice, you have two options to consider: open awareness or focused attention, illustrated on the opposite page.

Open awareness means you notice the thoughts that arise, but you don't engage. You just allow them to be there, without judgment. You sit with whatever comes up, coming back to your breath as you do so.

Focused attention means you determine a focus before you begin, coming back to that anchor every time your mind wanders (and it may wander a lot). This anchor could be your breath, the sounds you can hear, or your bodily sensations.

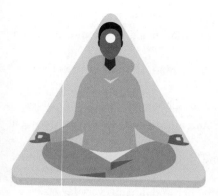

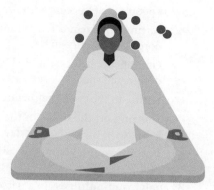

Open awareness

Watch the thoughts that arise in your mind. Allow them to come and go, but don't engage or judge

Focused attention

Focus on an anchor, such as your breath, the sounds you can hear, or your bodily sensations

If you'd prefer some guidance, consider trying out an app as your tool. Some popular choices are Insight Timer, Calm, Headspace, and Jabumind (which is specifically for classroom teachers).

If you know you like accountability, you could find a sitting group in your area or ask like-minded teachers to meet routinely. Many live guided mindfulness practices are offered virtually. I make this suggestion because practicing alone may seem daunting. Although you may find a solo practice useful as you progress on your journey, it's certainly not something you have to do.

After choosing your place, time, and tool, start with five minutes a day and build from there. Studies suggest 15-20 minutes a day is ideal. If you can't find that much time, don't abandon the practice. It's much more effective to sit for one minute each day of the week than to hold out for the "perfect" amount of time on the weekend. Build the habit first and increase the time as you can, rather than wait to build your habit until you achieve ideal conditions. We will never have ideal conditions. Teachers know better than anyone how the unexpected always happens.

In future chapters we'll work on creating intentions, goals, and plans, but for now, just try to find those five minutes. If you're worried about adding something else to your to-do list, consider taking an honest appraisal of how you spend your time during the day. See if there are any five-minute periods when you surf websites or zone out to a TV show, and consider replacing one of those periods with this practice.

Some people have success with practicing at moments such as these:

- Setting an alarm a few minutes earlier than usual in the morning, and doing the practice in bed.
- Getting up before the rest of the household and sitting quietly in a designated spot.
- Sitting in the car either before going into school or after leaving school.
- Shutting off the lights in the classroom and sitting at the desk during a break or at the end of the day.
- Putting your phone/book away and doing the practice in bed before falling asleep.

By applying mindfulness in a personal practice and during everyday tasks, we practice for the big game: the big game of life – and life as a classroom teacher. This leads us to practice option #3.

Practice option #3: school and classroom moments

Just as we're adding mindful awareness to mundane activities, in practice option #3 we add mindful awareness at strategic, sensible moments in our school day.

For example, can you take three deep, mindful breaths each time your students leave your classroom, or as they transition to different activities?

Can you get into the habit of feeling your feet on the ground when you begin each activity?

Can you practice making eye contact and acknowledging each student as they enter your classroom?

Can you commit to just eating your lunch, instead of working through your break and neglecting your most basic needs?

Can you take a moment for some fresh air or a little walk at lunchtime?

Try to find one practice you can commit to throughout your school day. And do your best to do that, today. We're trying to become aware of moments where mindfulness may be a natural fit. We'll create a formal classroom plan later in the book, but, for now, just become interested in experimenting with what might work for you, your current school schedule, and the students you're working with.

Practice option #4: deliberate self-care

Getting up early, sitting with no entertainment, putting the devices away, simply breathing – none of that sounds precisely like self-care, but I assure you it is. In the first three practice options, you're noticing yourself. You're paying attention to yourself. This is the first step in truly learning to care for yourself.

I've specifically added this fourth practice because I know teachers. Unless you're given permission to take some time for yourself in a more traditional "health and wellbeing" way, it may never happen. We know mindfulness is paying attention to what we're doing, when we're doing it. But we're going to extend this to paying attention to how we're caring for ourselves and creating a plan for things that nurture our souls.

A self-care plan and assessment can be found at www.teachingwell.life/pathbook. These will provide you with some data you can use to determine what you want to focus on in your deep dive into self-care. If anyone questions your motivations, simply explain that it's part of a school assignment. Smile and go take care of yourself for the time you've designated.

After taking the assessment and inventory, pull out the activities that speak to you and commit to adding something each day, each week, or each month, depending on the scope of your self-care plan. Have fun figuring out the activity that nourishes your soul but takes the least amount of time, energy, and effort. Can you do that activity each day?

For me, it's my first cup of coffee, specifically that first sip. I try to consciously take the first sip with mindful awareness and a little gratitude for all the people who worked for that coffee to arrive at my home. Just slowing down and homing in on that one moment is an act of self-care I look forward to each day. This practice costs little and takes no prior planning, other than making my coffee and bringing mindful awareness to that moment. To me, this is the perfect act of daily self-care.

My suggestion to you is to get into the habit of scheduling that self-care time. We've already established that external factors contribute to our stress and discontent in our classrooms, and that by working on our internal lives we can choose serenity over stress. The same principle applies to our personal lives. For self-care to happen, we must take the initiative and schedule it for ourselves.

Can you commit to scheduling some time in your calendar and making it happen? Can you keep the appointment with yourself, just like you would a good friend? Don't be afraid to take care of yourself. If you don't, who will?

Putting the practices together

We've run through a quick overview of what mindfulness practice can be and where you can practice. The reality is that you can practice anywhere, at any time, even when you're not doing anything (except sitting and breathing). My suggestion is to commit to doing one of the first three mindfulness practices each day. Perhaps you commit to five quiet minutes in the morning, or find a time during your school day to just breathe.

Try to work in a small self-care practice weekly, but commit to doing something that may take a little more planning within the next month. For me, it's working on a favorite hobby of mine: paper collaging and scrapbooking. When I was younger and didn't have a family beyond myself, it was easy to pull out the paper, glue, scissors, and paint when I felt like it. Now it's an exercise in deliberate self-care to ask my husband to watch our children while I create for an hour. It was hard to ask for that, but I needed to. It has nothing to do with teaching or my family, but that's the point. I need to do something that nurtures my soul in order to be my best self in my classroom and for my family. I encourage you to try it. See how you feel after putting the oxygen mask on yourself first. Do you feel a little lighter? A little freer?

When I teach my online mindfulness course, I suggest participants keep a 14-day mindfulness log (see www.teachingwell.life/pathbook for this resource) and try out different practices. At the end of that 14 days, some find that they like switching from practice to practice, sampling different things, like they would at a buffet. Others settle into one kind of practice and experience what that feels like day after day.

I ask you to remain curious and to put on your scientist's hat when trying these different techniques. Some will work for you, others will not be suitable. You may like some suggestions on some days and other suggestions on other days. Try to be gentle with yourself and the process as you experiment.

This still feels selfish...

I get it. But that's why you're committing to just a few moments a day, and after about 14 days you can check in with how you feel. If you need some support, I suggest joining an online accountability group or finding some like-minded teachers at school.

The only way to make this practice a habit is to make it a habit. And the only way to make it a habit is to do it every day. I've found creating a regular mindfulness practice similar to keeping up with an exercise routine. I'm more successful at sticking with a routine if I schedule something each day, whether that's a walk, a run, or a yoga session. Even if I only had a few minutes to walk, at least I did it. My brain remembers the effort and the experience. If I wait until I have time for a five-mile run before I do anything, then my brain won't get the experience of taking the time, putting on my sneakers, and moving away from my desk. However minor, the effort causes new neural pathways to be built that make my brain remember.

I've found that even practicing mindfulness for a minute is better than none at all. When my first son was born, I was exhausted (I still am at times) and sometimes I would set an alarm to just breathe for a minute. I was nervous about losing my personal practice when I had a child, but the most effective remedy against that was to simply do something each day and not wait for the perfect opportunity. If I had done that, I would probably still be waiting. The best time to start is right now!

It's no coincidence that the things that often fall by the wayside are those things we do for our own self-care. As educators, we can always find reasons to put others' needs before our own. We do that so often we might as well have a degree in it! So it's even more important for us to practice these moments of self-care habitually, because then excuses become a lot more challenging to find and ultimately believe. Accepting the Four Noble Truths of Teaching means we remember and remember again that much of our stress is caused by external factors. By focusing on our internal awareness and health, we can choose calm over chaos and serenity over stress.

By choosing to follow the Path of the Mindful Teacher, you're exploring things that will help you choose serenity over stress. One of those is to remember that it's self-care, not selfish. Even if you still believe, just a little bit, that you're being selfish, I ask you to put the doubt aside for 14 days and try to add a little self-care in the form of one of the mindfulness practices listed in this chapter. What do you have to lose by trying something different right now? You might get to the end of those 14 days and see a positive change in the way you feel.

Questions to ponder on the path

- What were your misconceptions about mindfulness?
- Now that you've read this chapter, how would you define mindfulness?
- What mindful practices are you going to add to your day? Week?
- If doubt begins to creep in, how will you remind yourself that self-care is not selfish?

Step into action

Try one (or all) of the following ways to add mindful moments to your day. Start a 14-day mindfulness log to keep track of your activities.

- Choose one way to add mindfulness to your daily activities and try to do this activity mindfully each day. This could be brushing your teeth, washing the dishes, driving to work, or eating a meal.
- Choose a place in your home (or somewhere else) that you can designate as your mindfulness practice space.

- Choose one way to add mindfulness to your school day. This could be three breaths between classes, or moving away from your desk for lunch, or taking a sip of water at the top of each hour.
- Complete the self-care assessment. Choose one way to add self-care to your day and one activity you'd like to do in the next week or month.

Featured five-minute practice: Body Scan

- Set your timer for five minutes.
- Focus on allowing your body to relax into the surface that's supporting you.
- Slowly scan your body from your head to your toes.
- Become curious about any sensation that arises and pulls your attention.
- Breathe into that space.
- As thoughts arise, note them and return to the body.
- Continue this cycle until the time is up.

Supplemental resources

Check out www.teachingwell.life/pathbook for more resources to accompany this chapter.

Part II.
The teacher's classroom

Explore how you can apply mindfulness to your classroom and how it can help you make choices, identify scripts, and build relationships

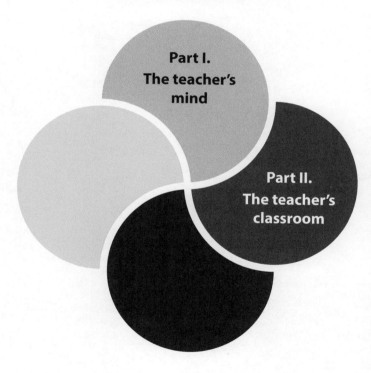

Part I.
The teacher's
mind

Part II.
The teacher's
classroom

Chapter 3.
Respond rather than react

Between stimulus and response there is a space. In that space is our power to choose our response. In our response lies our growth and our freedom – Unknown

Chapter objectives

You will be able to:

- Identify sensations, thoughts, feelings, and emotions.
- Analyze incidents of reacting vs incidents of responding.
- Develop strategies to defuse reactive situations.

I remember vividly how I felt when Angela looked into my eyes and told me she would absolutely not participate in the group discussion. In fact, she would stay right where she was, thank you very much. I remember the heat that rushed to my face, the prickly sensation along my shoulder blades. My heart began to beat more rapidly as my mind cataloged all the ways that this was going to end in disaster. One by one, the other students became much more interested in the interaction between Angela and me than in anything I had asked them to do. Now she had an audience. Now I was officially spinning.

"I'm not moving and this is so stupid." Angela raised her voice just enough for the other students to become virtually silent. Students always quieten down when these kinds of interactions occur.

"Angela, this is ridiculous. If you are not going to participate, go into the hallway." My voice was raised; I hoped the other students and Angela herself couldn't hear the quavering. I pointed my finger to the door.

Every time, it went something like this: Angela would leave the room, but not without pushing her seat back, shoving her materials on to the floor, walking off with a dramatic huff, and slamming the door. I would yell after her. Then I would go out into the hallway and give her a stern lecture. She would forcefully restate her intention of not doing the work and look away, fists and teeth clenched.

"You are being ridiculous," I would always say. "You know you can do this work. You're actually well advanced and really shouldn't even be in this class. What's your problem?"

But there was never any response. When Angela shut down, she wouldn't open her mouth to explain, discuss, or otherwise respond. Interestingly, she would come back into the classroom the next day without incident, seemingly over the issue of the previous day. She would greet me with a warm smile and a kind word. Sometimes we could spend weeks on amicable terms, but then something would happen and we would do this awful dance.

Roughly 90% of the discipline or defiance in my classroom came from teenage boys. For the most part, they just needed a time out and then they would come back into the classroom ready to get started. They were predictable. We had a known dance worked out, but with Angela all bets were off. I wasn't sure where I stood with her and that terrified me. If I'm being perfectly honest, I was thankful when she was gone from the room. The air seemed to lift. I could feel the energy change.

For some reason, it was difficult for me to see beyond her behavior. I was constantly on tenterhooks around Angela, but I didn't dig any deeper into why she was acting this way. I figured she just didn't like the class. Then, by accident, I started talking *to her* instead of *at her* – and everything changed.

It was the end of class. She was getting her stuff together more slowly on this particular day. I was rushing her a bit, because I didn't have any students the next period and had a lot of grading to get done. We hadn't had a particularly rough day, but I could tell something was bothering her. I was happy that it didn't seem to be me.

"Angela, what's going on?" I asked her calmly. Her eyes met mine. And then she started to talk, and I started to listen. She shared some things that were happening in the lunchroom.

A few days later, she stayed after class and shared some problems she was having with her mom.

A few days after that, she shared her fears about visiting her dad and stepmother for the holidays.

Each day, Angela shared a bit of herself in bite-sized doses. Of course, I listened for anything that was alarming, and tried to make sure I didn't become a counselor when my role was to be her English teacher. But it just seemed as if she wanted to let me in a little. I could feel her angst about finding her place in the school; about navigating friendships, relationships, and parents. It was clear she was trying to work out where she fit and how she fit, and that struggle is so raw and real for me. I could be her sounding board. I could just listen, if that was what she needed.

I was so proud of the way our relationship was evolving. Angela was a little less confrontational with me in class. She was still was a bit overbearing with her classmates, but it was getting better. There was progress. Then, one day, I asked her to do something and she reverted to her past behavior. She went right back to that defiant tone and the pushback when she had an audience.

But in that moment, *I did something different*. All the conversations Angela and I had shared came flooding back to me. Instead of seeing her as a kid who hated my class and clearly had undiagnosed oppositional defiant disorder, I saw her as a young person struggling to find her way. In that moment I saw her vulnerability, and realized that the behavior wasn't about me. In that moment I decided to flip the script.

I took a deep breath, made a little joke to her, and smiled. I let her have her space. I didn't engage with her the way she expected me to. I didn't meet her anger with anger; I met it with a warm smile and direct eye contact. My unexpected reaction meant she didn't have anything to push against. We continued the day without incident.

Angela continued to have outbursts. I continued to try to lighten the situation and she would quickly move on. I found that some of her objection to the work was that she was bored, and she lit up each time I suggested she go a little further with her analysis in writing, or that she read an additional short story to see if she could find the symbolism and theme in the piece. Soon I was assigning her work that was completed by my more advanced classes, because it was clear she was capable.

Our relationship was always a bit precarious, especially when she felt unsure of her place in school or felt she had to prove something. But the difference now was that *I wasn't taking it personally*. I had chosen to respond differently. I had taken the time to see the behavior as a product of something else.

Just before Thanksgiving, I asked the students to write a letter to someone they were grateful for. I suggested that they give their letter to the person over the holiday. Angela was finishing up her letter when the bell rang, and I wished her a great break as I walked back to my desk to get ready for my own break.

Angela walked over to my desk and extended her hand, which had a piece of paper in it. I didn't realize at that moment what it was, and looked at her quizzically. She said, "You told us to give the letters to the person we're grateful for, and I wrote my letter to you."

I smiled. Before I could say anything, she turned and walked quickly out of the room, not wanting to tarnish her reputation as one of the toughest girls in her grade. I opened the letter. Angela had thanked me for all the ways I had helped her as she adjusted to school and friends and family. She thanked me for listening. I got teary immediately. Really, all I had done was my job. I had responded, not reacted, to a student's behavior, and gotten to know that student as an individual, instead of just another troubled kid with something to prove.

I was heartened and saddened simultaneously. I was heartened because I had obviously helped Angela, but I was saddened by the thought of so many other students whom I hadn't helped. How many other students had I reacted to, because of my own overwhelming emotions, instead of responding to their behavior from a place of care and compassion?

Learning to respond

What I learned from that experience chimes with the Four Noble Truths of Teaching. My stress was caused by an external force (Angela), but only by paying attention to what I could control (my responses to her actions) was I able to move forward and develop a relationship with her.

I needed to explore how I felt when I was challenged in the classroom. I needed to bring mindful awareness to the physical sensations, thoughts, feelings, and emotions that I experienced when I was in my classroom. I could no longer just move through my day ignoring the signals my body was giving me. If I continued to do that, how many other Angelas would slip through the cracks? The only answer I could come up with was: too many.

At first, I wanted to beat myself up about what a terrible teacher I was and how much harm I'd inflicted upon all those other Angelas. I sat in that guilt and shame for a while (and still hang out there from time to time), but by applying mindfulness to my classroom experiences, I began to see it was a blessing that I was now paying attention to what was really happening with me and with my students.

That's what I want to offer you in this book: hope. Hope that through this practice you will begin to understand yourself better, leading to a change in how you show up in your classroom day after day. Nothing may change, but *you* will change, and that will make a difference in how you teach your classes, how you manage your stress, how you care for yourself, how you interact with parents, how you show up for meetings, and how you work with colleagues.

Now you've established your own daily mindfulness practice, it's time to explore the depth and breadth of the Path of the Mindful Teacher. The place where we seem to need it most is in our classrooms. Yes, we feel stress at home, with all our responsibilities and obligations. But at school a certain kind of stress is present, and it often has to do with the stuff that others bring into our classroom. Our students come to us with their own burdens, but remember: we can't control that. We can only control our own internal environment.

So, how do we slow down the pace of our reactions when the situation in our classroom is moving a mile a minute? How do we create space in an environment that is so complex? Well, we practice. One of the best things we can do is to keep track of our physical sensations, thoughts, feelings, and emotions for a period of time – I usually suggest a few days. Keep a piece of paper by your desk and note down what you experience. I call this a Mind/Body Connection Journal (find a template at www.teachingwell.life/pathbook) and it can do wonders for your self-awareness. I encourage you to be as judgment-free as possible as you write these things down. We're not at the point where we need to diagnose or fix anything; we're simply writing down what we observe, without judgment. For example:

- I felt tension in my chest when Bobby yelled out and didn't raise his hand.
- I yelled at Susie for being out of her chair again, because when she does that I feel disrespected.
- When this class came into the room, my shoulders tensed up.
- My breathing was shallow when I went over to see what Jimmy and Doug were doing in the corner.
- When I walked into the faculty meeting and looked around, I tensed up at the title of the presentation.
- When I heard the phone ring, my heart started to beat rapidly. My mind raced about who could be on the other line and what they could want.
- I heard the email ding and saw the principal wanted me to come to his office. My face became flushed and I felt faint. My knees were weak.

What are sensations, thoughts, feelings, and emotions?

Before we start to track our behaviors in the classroom, we must first understand exactly what we're tracking. So let's define these things individually.

Physical sensations

When I refer to sensations, I refer specifically to physical sensations in the body. For example, your face getting warm. Your hands tingling. Your fists clenching. Your stomach fluttering. Your shoulders tensing. Your heart beating more rapidly. Your breathing becoming shallow.

Sensations are anything you can identify physically. Many people find that they live much more in their minds than in their bodies, rarely addressing physical sensations, specifically pain or discomfort. So, although it seems straightforward, it may take some practice to really notice what you're feeling physically. One way to start noticing is to do a body scan practice (see page 44), perhaps during another activity like brushing your teeth or going for a walk. Notice what your body feels like when you're engaged in an innocuous activity. This can help you to more easily identify sensations when you're engaged in an altercation or a more heated situation.

Next, you might get into the habit of doing a quick body scan in your classroom before you begin your lesson, or before you walk into a faculty meeting or the lunchroom. Start at the top of your head and rest your attention on each body part as you scan down to your toes. You can choose to just pay attention, or to relax and release each part that feels tense or uncomfortable. By doing a simple scan regularly, you may start to notice patterns in how and when you tense up, or in your ability to relax depending on the circumstance.

Thoughts, feelings, and emotions

Although physical sensations often go unnoticed, it can be easier to identify a physical sensation than to identify your thoughts, feelings, and emotions. And then there's the issue of distinguishing between those three concepts.

This is the most straightforward way I've found to think about the differences:

1. **Thought**: a thinking process that happens in our minds by the coordination of various activities in our brains. Often this is experienced verbally as an inner monologue, or as visual images in a movie-like sequence or story.

2. **Feeling**: something happening externally is received by our five senses, then decoded by our brains.

3. **Emotion**: how we react or respond after experiencing the five-sense stimuli (the feeling).

Here's a simple example. You're walking down the street near an ice cream shop. You think, "Man, an ice cream would be so good," or you visualize eating the cone and imagine the taste (**thought**). You buy an ice cream and then taste it (**feeling**). You become happy (**emotion**).

And here's a classroom example. A student walks into the classroom after the bell rings. You immediately think about why he was late – "This kid has it in for me" – or you visualize him purposefully wasting his time on the way to your class (**thought**). You see him slam his books on his desk, whisper something to his friend, and then laugh (**feeling**). You become _____ (**emotion**).

I left the emotion blank because I don't know which emotion would arise for you. Would it be compassion? Anger? Annoyance? Disappointment?

We'll explore thoughts, feelings, and emotions more deeply later in this chapter, but for now you need to know that they are different ways for your mind to examine what's happening in the present moment. A problem can arise when the moment is filtered through past experiences, instead of responded to non-judgmentally. Think about that classroom example. Would your emotion be different if it was a certain student over another? Would you feel compassion for some students but annoyance at others?

Mindfulness practice makes us more aware of our thoughts, feelings, and emotions, and helps us avoid reacting to outside stimuli on autopilot. We instead practice *responding* mindfully and skillfully. Now you have some vocabulary to describe the concepts of thoughts, feelings, and emotions, you'll be able to keep a Mind/Body Connection Journal that will help you recognize those moments when your emotions are heightened.

Be as specific and descriptive as possible as you keep your journal. There's a saying: name it to tame it. What that means is that we must identify the thought, feeling, or emotion before we can actually do anything about it. We must label it as factually as possible, without judgment, before we can dig deeper into why we're reacting in a certain way.

So just write it down; we'll begin to analyze your notes later. These logs will be the basis for bringing full mindful awareness to your classroom. Without writing these things down and observing them, you may miss, skip, or avoid some of your "tells" when working with students. But when you recognize your seemingly automatic responses in certain situations, you can start to fortify your actions and begin to respond rather than react.

What does it mean to respond rather than react?

Responding rather than reacting is an especially important tool to have as a teacher. We are professionals who work with children day in and day out. If there's a group of people who are unpredictable with their emotions, it's children. Depending on their age, circumstance, background, life experience, hunger level, and home life, they may be a different student on a different day. From what we know about the brain, some of the unpredictability is because of rapid growth and development in their brains. This development, coupled with the trauma that many students are grappling with, can make for challenging situations.

Children often don't have the words or the tools to explain why they behave in a certain way, or feel a certain thing. And if we, as adults, don't know how to do that very well, how can we expect them to? If the students we work with don't have the tools to regulate their own emotions and behaviors, we must help ground them until they get the hang of it. That's why we must learn to respond mindfully to their behaviors, instead of reacting on autopilot to our own thoughts, feelings, and emotions.

The first step is to keep your Mind/Body Connection Journal for a few days (or more), so you can begin to see patterns in your physical sensations, thoughts, feelings, and emotions. After you analyze this journal for factual information and patterns, you can begin to add some "fail safes" into your classroom culture.

For example, when you feel a tightening in your chest, instead of just reacting to the stimuli, take a deep breath, pause, and relax the tightness. This is a way to respond instead of react. When the student who is "always late" walks in, get a late slip, put it on their desk, and find a moment to talk to them about what's preventing them from getting to class on time, instead of berating them in front of their peers. This is a way to respond to the immediate behavior and circumstance, rather than react out of habit.

Now, don't get me wrong – consequences for student behavior are necessary. Becoming a mindful teacher doesn't mean you become a pushover teacher. When I first embarked on this journey, I wondered that myself. Would this practice make me lose my edge? In lengthening my waiting and response times, would I suddenly become a target?

What I've actually found is that my responses have become, over time, a lot more reasonable, allowing me to meet the students where they are. When I look at each situation for what it is, instead of assigning all the student's past transgressions to the situation in the heat of the moment, I can keep my cool. I can meet the student in the present moment. I can get creative in how I find out why they're behaving in a certain way. I can be present with what's actually happening in my classroom. I can, to the best of my ability, provide a positive, healthy experience for all the students in my classroom. We will dive more deeply into how we can flip these reactive scripts in the next chapter, but for now the focus is on finding some ways to pause and respond to the actual situation, instead of reacting on autopilot.

Remember the Four Noble Truths of Teaching. The external stimuli (the behavior) is what's causing us stress, but we need to bring the focus back to what we can control – ourselves. Remember the words of the Serenity Prayer. Through consistent mindfulness practice, you will be able to discern what you have no control over and what you *do*. That will allow you to choose serenity over stress and calm over chaos.

I hope you're seeing that it all goes back to you, especially when you're working with students. The good news is that just as your stress is contagious, your serenity and calm can be too.

A note about 'negative' vs 'positive' experiences

As you keep track of your sensations, thoughts, feelings and emotions, you may have the initial tendency to label these as negative or positive. This is a very easy thing to do. Often we see a negative experience as one that causes us perceived pain, and a positive experience as one that causes us to feel good.

When we label experiences as positive or negative, our brains crave those we see as positive and seek to avoid the negative. Although it may not seem like it, this kind of labeling can become unhelpful. For example, if you label a feeling like sadness as negative then you may seek to bury your feelings of sadness, or feel shame when you experience this emotion. It's important to remember that sadness is neither positive nor negative. It just is.

Instead of looking at experiences through the lens of negative and positive, try more objective labels such as helpful or unhelpful; pleasant or unpleasant. Is this emotion helpful or unhelpful? Is it pleasant or unpleasant? Do I have a tendency to move toward pleasant ones and away from unpleasant ones? If this emotion is unpleasant, why? And what can I learn from noting and observing that experience?

As you keep your Mind/Body Connection Journal, you may also experience thoughts that elicit no real emotion. Those can be noted as "neutral." In the early days of noting your sensations, thoughts, feelings, and emotions, you may not really pick up on any neutral observations, but over time you may find you're mostly in a state of neutral.

Tying it all together

Remember my story about Angela? It was clear that I wasn't responding to her behaviors, I was reacting to them, and that was getting me nothing but an angry student. I wasn't grounding myself in a way that allowed me to skillfully handle the situation.

When I started to keep a Mind/Body Connection Journal, I quickly began to understand the "tells" that occurred in my body as physical sensations before

Angela and I had our blow-ups. I recognized the thoughts that raced through my head. I recognized the emotions that surged through my body. I began to focus on my breathing when I felt any of those twinges occurring. Just taking a few breaths – three, to be exact – created some space between stimulus and response. Instead of reacting, I responded. It didn't always happen perfectly. I didn't always notice my physical "tells," or sometimes I ignored them and reacted instead of responded. But in the moments that followed my reactions, I was *aware* of what had happened. Now, when I reacted, it seemed more of a choice and I chose to react more rarely than before.

I invite you to take stock of your emotions in your classroom for a few days. This investigation may not be easy, and you may not like all that you discover, but it will lay the groundwork on the Path of the Mindful Teacher and help you begin to choose serenity over stress and calm over chaos. This is our ultimate goal.

Questions to ponder on the path

- Which sensations, thoughts, feelings, and emotions cause you to react rather than respond?
- What can you do to defuse your self-identified reactive situations?

Step into action

- A Mind/Body Connection Journal template can be found at www. teachingwell.life/pathbook. Use it to help you track your physical sensations, thoughts, feelings, and emotions for three to five days.
- Reflect on your results, looking for patterns and "tells" that may indicate how you're going to react in certain situations.
- Create a plan for when you feel those "tells" emerging. Perhaps you could take three deep breaths or focus on your feet grounding into the floor.
- Continue your mindfulness practice, as established in Chapter 2, to gain more practice in working with sensations, thoughts, feelings, and emotions when the stakes aren't so high. Remember, we need to practice to do well in the "big game" that is our classroom.

Featured five-minute practice: Working with Thoughts

- Set your timer for five minutes (or more).
- Begin to focus on your inhales and exhales.
- Try to identify where you feel your breath the most. This is your anchor, your home base.

- When thoughts arise, "note" their presence but don't engage.
- After noting, return to the breath.
- Continue this cycle until the time is up.

Supplemental resources

Check out www.teachingwell.life/pathbook for more resources to accompany this chapter.

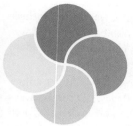

Chapter 4.
Identify scripts and blind spots

The only veil that stands between perception of what is underneath the desolate surface is your courage – Vera Nazarian

Chapter objectives

You will be able to:

- Analyze data from your Mind/Body Connection Journal to determine scripts and blind spots.
- Explore those scripts and blind spots.
- Determine effective methods to pause your reactions to scripts and blind spots.

The student walked through the classroom door late, once again. "So nice of you to join us," I said, as I huffed dramatically and reached for a late slip, or "pumpkin slip" as they're called at my school, because of their bright orange color. They are meant to stand out, to draw attention to the students who receive them.

I marched over and put it on his desk. Standing beside him as he scribbled his name on the slip, his signature making it official that he agreed he had been late, I could feel my temperature rising and my heart racing, although at the time I didn't really realize what was happening.

I won't mention this student's name, because he was one of so many, day after day, year after year. I met each late slip with a flurry of self-righteous anger that I sometimes did my best to stifle. At other times I felt justified. I was teaching these students a thing about respect. I was teaching them to think about others. I was teaching them to follow rules. Except, nothing ever really changed. The student would fill out the slip, but sooner or later they would be late again.

The same dance happened with pencils, materials, books. I would get angry, take the infraction personally, deduct points, take away privileges. But I was always left exasperated, frustrated, with a racing heart, a red face, and a clenched fist. I would deliver a lecture to the whole class, because I thought it was useful for everyone to hear. The trouble was, the kids who did what I asked weren't the ones who needed to hear the lecture, and the kids who needed to hear it really weren't listening. I cared much more about the rules, procedures, and protocols than those routine forgetters ever did.

In college, when we were taught classroom management, we learned that the classroom was something we had to control. When students did what they were supposed to (i.e. followed our agenda and plans), we got good marks in classroom management. This strategy relies on buy-in from students, and for the most part that may be forthcoming, but what about when it isn't? We often resort to raising our voices, delivering threats, and carrying out consequences – but to what end?

If it looks like you have your classroom management all worked out, is it really because the students are listening? Or are they going along with the arbitrary rules for fear of the consequences? What effect is had on those who are singled out and labelled as troublemakers? Have we ever asked ourselves, as teachers, where these expectations come from and who they benefit? Why do we cling so tightly to the way things are "supposed" to be?

When I really thought about it, I realized I was getting upset about the student's behavior but I wasn't digging into the reasons behind my reaction. This is the next step on the Path of the Mindful Teacher: identifying your scripts and then "flipping" them. Keep your Mind/Body Connection Journal close by and, in this chapter, we'll start flipping those scripts you're carrying around with you.

As Vera Nazarian suggests in the quote that opens this chapter, we need courage to dig beneath the surface and uncover what's really going on. Whoever thought getting to the heart of classroom management issues would take courage? I certainly didn't. My feeling was that if only the kids would listen, we would all be just fine. But when I finally paused and tuned into my own sensations, thoughts, feelings, and emotions, I realized my students were at the mercy of my own personal expectations and experiences. In order for anything to change, I would have to change.

In her book *Mindfulness for Teachers*, Patricia Jennings writes:

> *"We may assume that a student's behavior is conscious and intentional when it's more likely the result of poor regulation, trauma, or something going on outside of school. Our scripts may exaggerate our perceptions and blow things out of proportion. We may think a student misbehaves more frequently than he actually does. Finally, our scripts may lead to a tendency to act on unconscious biases without realizing it ... Attending mindfully to what is happening can help you recognize your emotional patterns and respond to them consciously rather than blindly reacting to emotionally provocative situations."*[2]

Remember my story about Angela in Chapter 3? After I started to identify my physical sensations, thoughts, feelings, and emotions in my interactions with Angela, I started to notice other unhelpful reactions to student behavior. If I'm being perfectly honest, it was a difficult realization. I had always aimed to be firm but fair, and to set high expectations for my students. I believed they needed to rise to my beliefs about what they could accomplish.

This turned out to be the wrong tactic with so many of my students, including Angela. When I began to respond instead of react to her behavior, I got to know Angela a little better. And as I learned more about her, I realized that many of the assumptions I made about her behavior – that she wanted to fit in, that she had something to prove, that she was purposefully defiant and not respectful – were stories I was making up in my head based on previous experiences of my own. I had preconceived notions about what student behavior should be, and when Angela (or anyone else) didn't meet those ideals, I was delivering consequences without much conversation.

As Angela and I began to interact more, I learned about her history and the obstacles she faced each day. Instead of cringing each time she walked into the room, I gave her a smile and a genuine welcome. Instead of shouting at her across the room, making her feel like she was under a microscope, I walked over and requested what I needed from her. When I started bringing mindful awareness to my own responses to her behavior, I needed to redirect her less and less often.

Learning to respond rather than react, and then learning to identify my scripts and blind spots, was more powerful than I could have ever imagined. It helped me choose serenity over stress and calm over chaos. It actually paved the way for my being able to stay in the teaching profession.

---

2. Jennings, P.A. (2015) *Mindfulness for Teachers: simple skills for peace and productivity in the classroom*, W.W. Norton & Company

Perhaps you've got this far along the Path of the Mindful Teacher and you're starting to feel that, for you, the only way to choose serenity and calm would be to leave the profession. If you're beginning to have that realization, I ask that you try to finish this book before altering your entire career trajectory. But if you give it some careful consideration and you still feel that way, well, then you have some choices to make. If you make the choice that's right for you, remember that's great for *everyone*, including your students, because everyone wins when we're happier and more fulfilled.

What are scripts?

We've all had experiences that have created emotional memories – experiences that have led us to harbor emotions in our body and in our mind. These emotionally conditioned scripts can resurface as strong negative emotions when activated by behaviors or circumstances.[3] Our perception of reality may be altered because the script is interfering with the way we see the current situation.

Scripts are usually developed as a necessity when we are children, in order to protect us. The problem is that even though we're no longer experiencing the same dangers, our body may continue the same response automatically. Not all emotional experiences will result in a script forming, but many of our scripts are hidden from us because they've become so ingrained.

If I revisit my story about Angela, it's clear that my script was that students should listen to teachers and "bad" behavior should be punished. My own parents set high expectations and instilled in me the importance of listening in school. In my early elementary years, I witnessed children who didn't behave being paddled. I certainly didn't want to be one of those students, so I sat up straight and did my work exactly as the teacher told us to.

My script is that all students should enter my classroom with that same level of respect, without exception. The problem is that students bring their own scripts to the classroom. When my script comes up against a student's script that the teacher is mean and doesn't like them, embedded over years of encountering similar teacher scripts, an eruption is inevitable.

Interestingly, the eruption doesn't have much to do with what's happening in the present moment. The teacher thinks the student is being outwardly defiant on purpose. The student thinks the teacher is picking on them. And if the teacher automatically assumes the behavior is defiance, based purely on the script that's running, no bridges can be built.

---

3. Ekman, P. (2007) *Emotions Revealed: recognizing faces and feelings to improve communication and emotional life*, Henry Holt

When we learn to slow down, and to respond instead of react to student behavior, we begin to notice if we have a script running. Remember: we can't control external factors, and that includes students and their own scripts. We can only control how we show up in our classrooms. It's far more effective to work with the present moment – grounding ourselves, taking a few deep breaths, meeting our students where they are – than to harbor anger, resentment, and old scripts that mean we can't see past student behavior to the individual person. We need to bring mindful awareness to our interactions with students, knowing that our script may rise to the surface. We may still come up against the students' own scripts, but if we can respond to their behavior instead of reacting, we may find that their scripts begin to shift a bit, allowing us to build deeper and stronger relationships in our classroom.

What are blind spots?

According to Mahzarin R. Banaji and Anthony G. Greenwald, authors of *Blindspot: hidden biases of good people*,[4] we all have hidden biases created by "a lifetime of exposure to cultural attitudes about age, gender, race, ethnicity, religion, social class, sexuality, disability status, and nationality ... our perceptions of social groups – without our awareness or conscious control – shape our likes and dislikes and our judgments about people's character, abilities, and potential."

As teachers, we may think that we don't have blind spots. We believe everyone is equal and should be treated the same, right? Of course, this is very true on the conscious level, yet we may be harboring blind spots without even thinking about them. We may teach in a community of students whose cultural or ethnic background is unfamiliar to us. We may believe students should make eye contact to show respect, but this is not the custom in some cultures. Blind spots are a particular kind of script that, in our current cultural climate, we should examine more thoroughly.

The biggest challenge when it comes to tackling our blind spots is that we may have no idea they are even present – they are hidden biases. We have a responsibility to try to expose them to ourselves. This can be really difficult work. It can be really painful work. But doing this work will allow us to be present in our classrooms and to see students *as they are*, instead of who we think they should be.

Remember: when we bring mindful awareness to our classroom situations, we bring a non-judgmental mind. We may not be able to change our scripts and

---

4. Banaji, M.R. & Greenwald, A.G. (2013) *Blindspot: hidden biases of good people*, Delacorte Press

blind spots, but we can move forward from a place of knowledge, choosing to recognize these scripts and blind spots so that we can respond to our students more mindfully. Now that we understand our own reactions, we can choose to do things differently.

Can scripts and blind spots be helpful?

Your scripts and blind spots probably were helpful in childhood, either to protect you or to help you fit into a certain community or group. They were probably a defense or survival mechanism for quite some time. Now that you're an adult, however, you have a choice to determine what remains helpful and what is now not so helpful. Bringing awareness to these scripts and blind spots will help you to work with them.

Perhaps you have a script that everyone should work hard and seek to achieve their best at any cost. This may have helped you through some difficult periods in your life. It may have taught you resiliency. It may continue to help you achieve. However, maybe it's not appropriate for you to automatically go to that script if a student isn't working to their perceived potential. Is it possible that there is more to the lack of effort than meets the eye? Is it possible to move beyond the script, considering what might be going on at this particular moment for this particular student, rather than writing them off as lazy or unmotivated? Is it possible to respond with curiosity rather than judgment?

Some blind spots helped you become part of and stay part of a community or family unit. This is why blind spots can be so insidious, pervasive, and confusing. They served a purpose, but now they may be keeping you from building relationships with people outside of your family, culture, or community. When you bring mindful awareness and light to your blind spots, you may uncover some that are uncomfortable. Be gentle with yourself. Having blind spots doesn't mean you're a bad person. Once you've uncovered them, you need to decide if they are worth maintaining because they have and continue to serve you well, or if they need to be addressed because they are detrimental to your relationships with others.

How can I flip my scripts?

As we learn to choose serenity over stress, part of the process is learning how to work with all the students who walk through our classroom doors, to the best of our ability. By growing our awareness of our scripts and blind spots, we become aware of our tendencies and our automatic responses. As we learn to respond rather than react to triggering situations, we practice seeing things through the lens of the present moment. And if we look at each situation with fresh eyes, we begin to change our scripts and see our blind spots.

On the next page is a Flip the Script Journal template. If you downloaded the Mind/Body Connection Journal template from www.teachingwell.life/pathbook, it should look familiar, because it's the same template with an extra column.

The Flip the Script Journal asks you to consider the moment in time that's causing stress or chaos, and to see if you can flip your script, allowing you to take the situation less personally. To further assist you, I've included examples of teacher scripts and how the teacher was able to flip these scripts.

Flip the Script Journal

1. Write down the facts of a situation (classroom or otherwise) that really "grinds your gears" or brings an emotional response. Try to think of actual moments, not just a representation of them.
2. Write down where you can feel physical sensations during this moment.
3. What thoughts are running through your head?
4. What is the script/message/tape running through your mind at this moment (this is usually a generalized conclusion)?
5. How can you "flip this script"? How can you look at this situation in the moment, rather than looking at it through what your script says is happening?

1. The facts	2. Physical sensations	3. Thoughts/emotions	4. What's the script?	5. How can I flip the script?
EXAMPLE: A student told me upon arrival today, after having a snow day yesterday, that he did not do his homework because he was sick.	Closed my mouth tightly, walked away, felt annoyed.	Annoyed, disbelief. I felt that he was fibbing.	The script is: "Of course he's going to say he didn't feel well and that's why he didn't do it. He probably never even thought about it or opened his bookbag before entering the classroom today."	When I walked away from the student, I realized I was not giving his story any credibility. So, a few seconds later I went over to his desk and asked about his illness; he described a headache/cold. I told him I was glad he was feeling better and to please complete the assignment tonight for partial credit. What I realized is that at least with rapport with this student, maybe he'll consider completing his assignment tonight.

Can mindfulness practice help us flip our scripts?

Mindfulness practice can be a very powerful way to recognize and work with scripts and blind spots. It helps us become aware of the present moment without judgment – and the "without judgment" part can be the most difficult when it comes to scripts and blind spots. We often want to judge and shame ourselves for our behaviors and biases.

Before practicing mindfulness, you may have felt guilty about yelling at a student or being impatient with an entire class. You may have felt unhappy about accusing a student of not paying attention or sending another student to the hallway for a minor infraction. When we practice mindfulness, we observe our reactions in the present moment and learn to pause – hopefully, we'll be able to respond more appropriately the next time the opportunity presents itself. Bringing mindful awareness to your classroom helps you see more of the picture. The student who is openly defiant each day is probably not doing this to you because he's a jerk. With mindfulness, you can slow down and treat this student as an individual, not as a character in a script that plays in your mind on autopilot.

Practicing mindfulness outside the classroom and at routine times through the school day will help you recognize your triggers – those things you wrote down in your Mind/Body Connection Journal. This may take the power and emotion out of your scripts and turn a light on your blind spots, essentially flipping the script on your automatic reactions. This frees you to work with the situation as it truly is. Of course, this is not an overnight fix. There will be times when reactions happen and all that we've learned about ourselves flies out the window. We will address how to work with those realities in a later chapter.

One thing that I found difficult about this process was the guilt I felt about some of the scripts and blind spots I uncovered. I had always thought I was a good person who wanted the best for my students. When I began to work with the realities of my scripts and hidden biases, I felt terrible about all the students I may have harmed through my automatic reactions. Nevertheless, I urge you to move forward with this work even if it's a little or a lot uncomfortable.

A quote that really resonates with me on this path is, "You only know what you know." Can you apply this quote to your realizations? In the days when I was unaware of the scripts and blind spots driving me, I lacked the knowledge and power to change my behaviors. But once I paused and started to dissect these scripts and blind spots, I knew differently. I didn't have that excuse to fall back on any more and I was able to work on flipping my scripts. I was the solution. This is both empowering and frightening – with great power comes great responsibility.

Tips for identifying/working with scripts

- When you feel a strong emotion, pay attention to the thought patterns associated with the emotion.
- Look more closely. Is there something "behind" the emotion that causes you to be uncomfortable? If the answer is yes, your response may be the result of a script rather than what's actually happening in the present moment.
- Continue recording in your Mind/Body Connection Journal and Flip the Script Journal to see if you can recognize patterns in your difficult emotions.

If you still want to move forward with this work despite its potential difficulty, I applaud you. You are about to embark on a process that may change the way you see yourself, your classroom, and your world. If you want to walk the Path of the Mindful Teacher, this is the way toward choosing serenity over stress and calm over chaos.

Mindful observation through your Mind/Body Connection Journal and Flip the Script Journal is the process by which you'll learn about your scripts and blind spots. Your journal will give you the data you need. Look at the data you've already recorded. Are there patterns in your thoughts? Are you assuming things about particular students? Are you thinking particular things before reacting to their behavior? If you haven't written down those kinds of details, continue recording for a few more days. Remember that you're in data-collection and judgment-free mode. You are simply observing yourself and making notes.

Once you have your data, try to identify patterns and see if there's something "behind" your reactions. If the same categories of students continually appear in the journal or similar situations arise throughout the day, this may indicate scripts or blind spots. When you spot those patterns emerging, simply ask yourself, "What could this be about?" and see if anything becomes clearer.

Scripts about yourself

One thing to really be on the lookout for is the script you may have about your own worthiness and ability to take time for yourself. This probably won't show up in your Mind/Body Connection Journal, but it may reveal itself when you prepare to take five minutes to practice mindfulness and the script arises that you should be doing something else. Or when you want to go for a short walk at lunchtime and the script arises that you're being selfish – you have papers to grade and things to do.

This script is insidious and, if not kept in check, can harm you and your progress. The script that taking time for yourself is selfish, that putting everyone else's needs first is best, or any other variation on that script, will keep you from choosing serenity over stress not only in your classroom but also in your life. It's important to acknowledge that this script is real; then you can move forward into actions *today* that will help your health and wellbeing.

It may be eye-opening to learn about the scripts and blind spots that govern your interactions with students, but it can be even more powerful when you uncover the scripts you tell yourself about your own worthiness and importance. We need to learn how to flip the script on this tape running through our heads, because it will ultimately keep us from choosing serenity over stress and walking the Path of the Mindful Teacher. Again, this work may seem simple, but it's not always easy.

As teachers, we are in a caring profession and this care may have spilled over into our families, friendships, and communities. This is not a bad thing. It's an incredible gift to be able to give so much to so many. However, being in a caring profession means you're also responsible for caring for yourself. So, treat any scripts that arise about yourself just like the classroom scripts you're uncovering. Ask yourself:

- Is there a story behind that script?
- Is the script true?
- Does the script serve me and my purpose of choosing serenity over stress?

You can explore the answers to those questions in your Mind/Body Connection Journal.

Will this step be worth it?

The short answer is a resounding YES! It won't be easy, but it will be worth it. The nonjudgmental data you collect in your Mind/Body Connection Journal and Flip the Script Journal will help you start to uncover your own hidden biases or blind spots. Because these beliefs may be ingrained or difficult to see, it may take some time to see how they manifest in your classroom. Think about your classroom as a laboratory. Try to practice mindful awareness in situations where these blind spots may be hiding. Bring your full attention to the present moment, holding on to your knowledge and awareness of the blind spot.

Remember, this thinking has become ingrained over years. It may not be remedied overnight. In fact, it's less about changing scripts or blind spots, and more about being mindful of them, so they don't get in the way of your work with students. You can better meet students' needs if your "stuff" isn't muddying the waters.

The more present you are in the classroom, the less opportunity there will be for your scripts and blind spots to arise. Paradoxically, by acknowledging them, they may start to disappear – or at least they won't have such a profound impact on your interactions. As we learned in Chapter 3 about our thoughts, feelings, and emotions, you have to name it to tame it.

In my case, I still hand out the pumpkin slips when a student arrives in my classroom late, but without so much glee and condescension. Rather, I ask the student to write a note about why they were late. Then I take the slip and we discuss it at the end of class. Sometimes I turn them in, sometimes I just hold on to them. It's no longer all or nothing. And the script that was running beneath the surface? The one that told me everyone who doesn't comply with the rules is disrespectful and should suffer the consequences? Well, I've had the courage to explore that script and let it go as an absolute rule. Sure, it sounds in my ear from time to time, but more often than not I see the student before me and hear them out, rather than reacting on autopilot.

Questions to ponder on the path

- What are the typical classroom behaviors or school scenarios that cause you to react?
- What are your prevalent scripts and blind spots?
- Where do these scripts and blind spots originate from?
- How have these scripts and blind spots been helpful and unhelpful to your students, your classroom, and/or yourself?

Step into action

- Build on your Mind/Body Connection Journal for three to five days by adding the Flip the Script column.
- Look at the data and explore what may be behind the script or blind spot.
- Experiment with techniques that can help you pause and flip the script when reactive situations occur.

Featured five-minute practice: RAINN

- Set your timer for five minutes.
- Focus on a moderately difficult incident (perhaps even a script you have).
- Recognize what's happening in your body/mind at this moment.
- Accept that this is happening and take a few breaths.
- Investigate: pause and notice your thoughts.
- Nurture: put your hand on your heart (or do some other comforting action), acknowledging what you have control over and what you don't.

- Next: what can your next action be to move you in a positive direction?
- Take a few breaths. Continue this cycle until the time is up.

Supplemental resources

Check out www.teachingwell.life/pathbook for more resources to accompany this chapter.

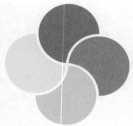

Chapter 5.
Create a safe 'container'

There is really nothing more to say – except why. But since why is difficult to handle, one must take refuge in how – Toni Morrison

Chapter objectives
You will be able to:
- Recognize your current methods for creating a safe classroom container.
- Develop a plan for deliberately building a safe container.
- Determine how mindfulness can support you to do this.

When I first started teaching, I thought "getting to know you" activities with new students were great at the beginning of the year. They allowed me to easily craft some opening lesson plans and gave me time to actually learn the students' names.

These activities included Two Truths and a Lie, interviewing one another, giving a speech, coloring a mandala, deciding which colors represented them and why, and writing an "I am" poem. The students brainstormed the behaviors they wanted to see in the classroom and the behaviors they didn't want to see. They formed small groups and discussed these ideas, producing a little visual depicting their consensus. We drew up a class contract that everyone signed, and we hung it at the back of the classroom to remind us of the behaviors we had agreed upon.

These were good exercises, but my intention was really unclear and not at all deliberate. To begin with, I did these activities because I was told in college to do them. I did them because I'd always done them. I didn't always think much of them: some years I thought, "This is so silly. Doesn't every student want to feel respected or not bullied?" Or, "How many more students are going to say the color that most strongly represents them is red, because they're full of energy?"

At one point, I considered dropping the introductory activities altogether. The way I thought about it, these activities only benefited me. They were a way for me to get to know my students, but I thought I could get to know them just as well through interacting with them in class. I primarily taught ninth grade and thought the majority of the students already knew each other. Furthermore, I figured that the kids thought the activities were silly and I should just get on with the academics.

As you read this, you may be shaking your head, thinking, "Wow, you really didn't get it, Danielle." You would be right, but luckily I do now. These activities are for the teacher *and* the students. In my first 10 years of teaching, I just thought it was nice for everyone to know those things about each other. But what I now know is that these first few days of class are some of the most important of the year.

In these early days, I'm not just getting to know names, interests, and personalities. I'm also building a little classroom community, a refuge, a safe "container" for my students. It was only once I started to study the epidemic of stress in the classroom and the trauma many students carry with them that I understood how essential it is to build a safe classroom container.

Some of you may be rolling your eyes at my ignorance over so many years of teaching, but I want to be honest. I did all the activities, and they worked in some regard, but I didn't proceed in a purposeful way toward building this safe container as the year progressed. Most of my students probably would have said that my classroom didn't harbor too many bad feelings and that it felt relatively safe. I think that may just have been out of luck, not because of any special ability of mine to cultivate community.

Then I got the class that almost made me quit teaching. You know the class. I vividly remember sensing that something was terribly amiss when one student interrupted me during my opening remarks in the first lesson. He had the whole class laughing and I was thrown off my game. On the first day, the students usually sat at attention, sometimes boredom. "This student obviously didn't get the memo," I thought to myself as he immediately sought out my attention – and not in a good way. And I didn't respond to his interrupting me in a kind tone. It was only five minutes into class, the "getting to know you" activities hadn't even started, and already I was yelling across the room at a student.

Eventually, we went through the motions of completing the activities, but there was no real attempt from me to get to know the class. As the weeks went by and the course rolled on, I forgot which kids liked hunting and who played soccer. As they butted heads and I yanked them out of the classroom for being rude, disrespectful, and mean, I didn't seek a resolution or try to help them find common ground. When one student returned from a three-day suspension for fighting another student in my classroom, I simply created a barrier of students and desks between the two kids and crossed my fingers that it would all be OK. I never considered how the students sitting between the two may have felt. Could I have triggered something in them, being caught in the middle like that? I'm embarrassed to say that it never even crossed my mind.

It was not my finest hour (or school year). I had no real plan. I had no real solution. My room wasn't big enough to separate all the problem students, but it was too big for me to keep an eye on what everyone was doing.

I survived that year, barely. Many of those students came back to my classroom as they progressed through the school, laughing at how bad they had been and how they would get me going. I was baffled, because they seemed to have built a rapport with me but to have no interest in building a working community with each other. I chalked that year up to an anomaly and crossed my fingers that I wouldn't get a class like that again. But I knew I needed to do something different.

This was the precise time that mindfulness practice first became a part of my life. I was starting to deliberately slow down and practice being present in my life outside school, and some of this rolled over into the way I interacted with students in my classroom. Of course, I eventually got another doozy class, but the experience wasn't the same this time, because I wasn't the same.

Remember Angela? Yes, it was Angela's class that challenged me this time, but I was more prepared and more grounded. I didn't yet have the Four Noble Truths of Teaching, or know that I could choose serenity over stress and calm over chaos. I hadn't yet discovered the Path of the Mindful Teacher. But what worked with that class was that I intentionally tried to build a safe classroom container. As echoed in Toni Morrison's quote at the start of this chapter, the key question wasn't *why* these students needed a safe container or what they had experienced in their past. The key question was *how* I was going to create this safe container for them.

Through the little bit of practice I had with mindfulness, I began to respond rather than react. I realized that much of the student behavior wasn't about me. The scripts and blind spots were there, but I could see them. Now that I knew these things, it was up to me to do something different. I felt up to the challenge and, for some reason, I realized that the way to survive this class – and perhaps even to thrive – was to work on building a classroom community. But I needed to *really* build one, not just do some "getting to know you" activities and then forget all that was learned.

What we'll be exploring in this step on the Path of the Mindful Teacher is how to be *deliberate* in building this container. You're a caring person and your students will feel that, but what happened to me was that my caring wasn't enough – especially when the students weren't doing what I wanted them to do, and when they weren't capable of being respectful to each other.

What is a safe classroom container?

Traditionally, a classroom is a place where students gather physically, surrounded by the same four walls. I'd like to broaden our definition of a classroom to a "container" where you reach your students together. This could be in-person, virtually, or in hybrid conditions. Some of you may never meet your students in real life, but you'll be able to reach them through the wonders of technology. The container is where everyone comes together, regardless of whether or not we're in the same physical space.

When so many students come to us having experienced trauma, it's so important that our classroom container is a predictable space. In order to learn, children must feel safe, and in order to feel safe, many children find comfort in routine. If the general routines and procedures are known and followed by everyone, this creates space for learning, fun, and exploration.

It's likely that you already have these routines and procedures in place, but are you consistent from the first day of school to the last? Do some students follow the routines, but not others? Do you accept some behaviors on some days, but fly off the handle on others? Are some students always under your watchful eye, while others get away with things behind your back?

Research shows that our brains can be hijacked by stress. According to Marc Brackett and Christina Cipriano of the Yale Center for Emotional Intelligence:

> *"Chronic stress, especially when poorly managed, can result in the persistent activation of the sympathetic nervous system and the release of stress hormones like cortisol. Prolonged release of this and other neurochemicals impacts brain structures associated with executive functioning and memory, diminishing our ability to be effective educators and undermining student learning."*[5]

When we're in the fight, flight, or freeze mode of response, which can happen very easily in stressful situations, we're not able to put the stress aside and let the learning process happen. So, we need to alleviate students' heightened stress

---

5. Brackett, M. & Cipriano, C. (2020) Teachers are anxious and overwhelmed. They need SEL now more than ever. *EdSurge*, www.edsurge.com/news/2020-04-07-teachers-are-anxious-and-overwhelmed-they-need-sel-now-more-than-ever

responses as quickly as possible so that real learning can take place. Remember, the Four Noble Truths of Teaching say we must be mindful of external factors, but work on our own internal responses in order to find a more balanced teaching life. What that means in this context is creating a safe container where students can leave their stress at the door.

In addition to general rules concerning leaving the classroom, going to the bathroom, arriving late, needing a paper, forgetting a pencil, and asking a question, creating a safe container can also include routines for your class flow. Do your days follow a similar pattern? Are there days or times for certain activities? Consider whether there are places where you can create a more consistent and deliberate routine. You may be surprised at how this supports your own grounding and planning.

It's been so helpful for me to create a specific order in which my class flows. I always start with a Silent 60, which is 60 seconds of quiet sitting. Students can put their heads down, close their eyes, or stare into space – I just ask that they are quiet and respectful of others. After 60 seconds, we start class. It's a great transition, allowing me and my students a bit of a buffer between classes. Although this could be considered a mindfulness practice, I don't really set it up that way – I just consider it a mini-break.

How to build a safe classroom container

Creating a safe container involves establishing rules, procedures, and routines that everyone understands and can adhere to. Creating a safe container involves being present with how you're feeling and with how your students are responding or interacting with you and one another. With appropriate procedures and routines in place, students can leave some of their worry at the door and become more fully engaged with the lesson and the learning opportunities. Even if students are learning virtually, we can create a safe classroom container for them. Many of these techniques are adaptable and can be used regardless of our physical container.

It's likely that you have some or most of these procedures in place already, but perhaps you want to be more deliberate about your intentions. If you're still unsure or want some additional suggestions, here are some easy ways to build a safe classroom container.

Establishing rules and procedures

1. **Create a classroom contract.** Ask students to write down the behaviors they want to see in the classroom and those they don't. Hold small group discussions and then a large group discussion. As a class, decide on general

rules of behavior that everyone can agree to and what that behavior looks like. Ultimately, the contract should be signed by all students and displayed so it can be referred to throughout the class. If the contract is not being followed, this should be pointed out and discussed with individuals or the entire group, depending on the situation.

2. **General class procedures.** Established routines are necessary for general procedures, such as going to the bathroom, arriving at class late, forgetting a pencil, asking a question, requesting a worksheet, and forgetting homework. You may want to brainstorm your own expectations about how these procedures and routines will be handled before the school year starts, then go over these expectations and procedures with your students. Some of the procedures can be co-created, but others will be up to you to establish. Depending on the age of your students, you may want to use signs, songs, or routines to aid transitions or remind the class of your expectations.

CALM classroom framework

If you're in need of a simple framework to help you build relationships, move content learning forward, find a little space to breathe, create a consistent routine for you and your students, and provide them with tools for practicing mindfulness, while building social-emotional learning (SEL) into your already full schedule, then look no further.

The CALM classroom framework was inspired by the SEL 3 Signature Practices Playbook[6] from the Collaborative for Academic, Social, and Emotional Learning (CASEL), the University of Pennsylvania's BDA framework,[7] and my own work in bringing mindful moments to the classroom through Teaching Well. The framework has four distinct sections that allow teachers to integrate touch points and check-ins throughout a class and/or the school day:

Caring Openings.

Actions Throughout.

Last Thoughts.

In the Moment.

---

6. https://schoolguide.casel.org/uploads/2018/12/CASEL_SEL-3-Signature-Practices-Playbook-V3.pdf

7. Found in Botel, M., & Botel Paparo, L. (2016) *The Plainer Truths of Teaching, Learning and Literacy*, Owl Publishing

Caring Openings

Provide time at the start of each class for a brief check-in, settle-in, or community-building activity. This daily routine or ritual provides you and your students with clear expectations and a chance to pause before beginning the lesson. Here are five ways to provide Caring Openings.

1. **Silent 60.** Ask students to sit quietly and comfortably as you give them 60 seconds to reset and get ready for learning. This is a great (and easy) way to start a class. Add-ons can include: focusing on sounds or breathing while sitting; body scan (from the top of the head down to the toes); and focusing on the five senses (ask students to identify something for each sense).

2. **The Power of Listening.** Ring a bell, a wind chime, or anything else that creates a long trailing sound. Ask the students to listen and silently raise their hand when they can no longer hear the sound. After the sound ends, ask the students to focus on the other sounds they can hear for the next minute. When the minute ends, ask each student to tell you what sounds they heard.

3. **Weather Check.** Ask students to sit quietly for a minute and think about how they could use weather analogies to describe how they're feeling. Depending on the age of your students, you may want to give an example the first time you try this – "I'm feeling sunny because I was able to get a little extra sleep this morning." You may want to circle back with those who express difficult weather "patterns."

4. **One Minute for Good.** Ask students to take a few deep breaths and invite them to put their heads down if that's more comfortable. For the next minute, ask them to think about the things they're grateful for, or that bring them happiness.

5. **Song, Image, Story, Quote.** Start each class with a themed song, image, story, or quote that can inspire discussion, get students thinking, increase engagement, or open up a big idea that you'll be discussing in class.

Actions Throughout

These interactive and reflective practices serve as check-ins for students (and teachers). They can be anchored to content or implemented at certain transition times throughout the class or day. Deliberately using a variety will help you reach most students on most days. Here are five ways to provide Actions Throughout.

1. **Think, Ink, Pair, Share.** After posing a question or introducing a big idea, allow Think and Ink time in which students can write down a personal response. Then they can pair up with a peer and share their thoughts more comfortably and readily.

2. **Partner discussions/large group share**. Instead of starting with large group discussions, scaffold with smaller groups and then transition to a larger group. Students will have more confidence in their answers if they are first allowed to share and support one another in pairs.

3. **Individual think time (deliberate wait time)**. After asking a question, pause to allow students to process their thoughts, instead of just calling on the first raised hand. Encouraging students to write their initial thoughts down as you pause for a designated amount of time can allow them to arrive at more complete answers.

4. **Brain breaks**. At designated intervals, or when you deem necessary, allow students to take a brain break. This could be a movement break or a slow-down break. These moments are deliberate and provide an opportunity for the students – and you! – to regroup.

5. **Mindful transitions**. Encourage movement between activities to take place in a mindful way, with students bringing total awareness to the transition. Ask them to pay attention to how many steps they take, the sounds they can hear, and the supplies they carry with them as they transition from one activity to another, or from one place to another.

Last Thoughts

Closing each class or school day in an intentional way is an opportunity to highlight individual or shared understanding, to set next steps or future goals, and to make connections or ask questions. Below is a list of Last Thought sentence stems to help you check students' understanding and address any questions they may have.

1. Something I learned today...

2. I am curious about...

3. I am looking forward to tomorrow because...

4. Something I'll do next...

5. Something I still question...

In the Moment

You can use these quick and discreet mindfulness practices when you feel a certain emotional response in class or throughout the day, when you notice your students need a reset, and at pre-planned times in your schedule.

1. **Three breaths**. At intervals during the day (between classes, for example), or when you feel emotions or tension rising, simply take three breaths. This is a great way to create a little space between a stimulus and a potential reaction.

2. **Centering**. When you're standing in front of a class, pay attention to how your feet feel on the ground. Really plug into being grounded and present. Take a moment to pause before getting started with the lesson.

3. **Breath awareness**. When you feel a stressful moment arising, bring awareness to your breath. Get curious about what happens to your breath in these situations. Don't hesitate to explain to your students what you're doing – modeling this breathing practice during times of stress can be really valuable to students.

4. **Body scan**. Between classes or at lunchtime, do a quick body scan, checking in with any place where you feel good or are holding tension. Try to bring some awareness and relaxation to the areas that are tense.

5. **Heartfulness practice**. Throughout your day, repeat the following phrase to yourself: "May I enjoy wellbeing, happiness, and peace." As students walk into class, as you navigate the busy hallways, or as you pass a difficult colleague, silently say, "May you enjoy wellbeing, happiness, and peace." You may want to teach students these phrases, so they have a tool for sending care to themselves and others during difficult times – or just because.

The CALM framework can be adapted whether your classroom container is four walls, a computer screen, or a bit of both. Get creative, try something, and see what happens.

Building relationships in your classroom

Once you've established rules and a routine, there will be more space for relationship-building in your classroom. That's not to say that everyone will get along perfectly, or that you'll no longer have classroom management problems. But by being deliberate about structures and expectations, and holding everyone accountable, you can more easily build relationships with your students – and they with each other. And, of course, the better the relationships within your classroom, the more easily you'll be able to choose serenity over stress and calm over chaos.

This is why creating a safe classroom container is so necessary to reduce our stress levels. "Getting to know you" activities may seem trite, but they are precisely the building blocks needed for meaningful relationships. Go beyond the basic ice-breakers with the following activities.

Regular class meetings

If you wrote and agreed upon a class contract at the beginning of the course, then a class meeting is a perfect way to make sure it's being upheld. You can discuss changes with the class, as well as any problems with the weekly routine or the flow of the day/course.

Class meetings can also be an opportunity to check in about the students' day or week. They can be a time to debate an idea or talk about an upcoming quiz or test. There should be a general meeting agenda, but it doesn't need to last more than 15 minutes. These circle activities help kids feel safe and listened to, so make sure a procedure is in place regarding who can speak when and for how long.

Mindful listening and communication skills

Class meetings are a perfect time to teach the importance of mindful listening and mindful communication. You can practice both these concepts and reinforce the skills when students are working in groups and engaging in debates or discussions, large and small.

These skills are important in school, in relationships, at work, and throughout the students' lives, so they're worth taking some time to develop. As technology and social media vie for our students' attention – and ours, for that matter – it's even more imperative that we teach them how to pay attention and effectively communicate with us and each other.

Practice mindful listening by asking the students to listen and count the different sounds they can identify inside and outside the classroom. A discussion could arise about how sounds are around us all the time, even though we don't really hear them; it may be eye-opening for students to discover that "silent" isn't always silent. Of course, this practice isn't going to turn them into mindful listeners overnight, but the point is to bring awareness. Make a game out of trying to hear the clock tick when others are talking, or trying to hear what the teacher next door is teaching.

Mindful communication can also be taught or introduced in class meetings. It's an extension of this mindful listening practice and is such a powerful tool for students. Mindful communication is simply paying attention to what someone else is saying, *really* listening to them, then responding appropriately.

One exercise that I use is called Partner Practice, adapted from a Mindful Schools[8] activity. Students are paired up: Partner A tells a story for a minute or two; Partner B simply listens. When time is called, Partner B summarizes the story and tries to guess why Partner A chose to tell that story. Was it to entertain? Did they need advice? Were they feeling irritated? Did they just want someone to listen? Partner A tells Partner B if they were right, and answers any questions that Partner B might have. Then the two switch roles.

---

8. www.mindfulschools.org

At the end, they could discuss which aspect they enjoyed more: listening or speaking. They could also comment on whether they listened well enough to identify what their partner needed from them as a listener. Finally, they could share their experience of trying not to interrupt or interject with their own opinion.

By teaching students mindful listening and mindful communication, you'll create a safer, more cohesive classroom container. To a casual observer, nothing really appears to have changed, but you've altered the dynamics within your classroom.

Kindness and compassion

With so many students experiencing trauma in their lives outside school, they may not have a lot of opportunity to build their self-worth. Participating in compassionate acts, large and small, will boost their positive feelings and that can translate into changes in other areas of their lives. When students practice being kind to others, it can really fill them with pride and joy.

In the month of December, I sometimes hold a Kindness Challenge where everyone is encouraged to do one nice thing throughout the day. It could be as simple as holding a door open, saying goodbye to the bus driver, or even paying for the coffee of the person behind them in the queue. We write our kind acts on the board and add to them each day.

I also get the students to pick the name of a classmate from a hat: throughout the week, they have to do one kind thing for that classmate, anonymously. At the end of the week, it's revealed who had which classmate and the kind thing they did for them. In a non-threatening way, this exposes the students to how it feels to do good for others.

A more involved kindness activity that I do with my older students is to have them visit an elementary school to read with the children. The elementary kids love it and the older students feel like rock stars. They don't normally believe me when I say they'll feel such a sense of pride after reading to little kids, but they do. It's one of the best things I've ever implemented. It shows that the more we get our students to do estimable things, the more esteem they will develop.

When we talk about kindness and compassion as skills to learn, students can be less apprehensive. If they already feel safe in your classroom thanks to the consistent procedures, treatment, and flow, they may feel comfortable enough to try some of these new things and learn how good it feels to be kind and compassionate to others.

Learning about strengths

From a young age, we're encouraged to improve upon our weaknesses. If we aren't "good" at math, then we should get tutored. If we aren't "good" at another skill, we should try harder and spend more time practicing. Research suggests that by only focusing on improving weaknesses, we may be overlooking opportunities to teach our students very empowering things about who they are. According to a study, these strength building activities have been around for quite some time:

> *"As early as 1830, Froebel designed the first kindergarten to elicit the active power or strengths of children. In the 20th century, Binet's ... work was dedicated to enhancing the skills of students and to addressing deficits, not solely remediating problems. Hurlock's (1925) seminal work highlighted the finding that praise of students' work has a more powerful effect on performance than criticism of students' efforts."[9]*

So many of our students have been told that they're bad or no good. If we teach them about their strengths, they'll begin to learn a different truth about themselves and this may shift the dynamic in the classroom, especially if there are opportunities for them to utilize their strengths. Helping them to also recognize their classmates' strengths will encourage a respectful classroom dynamic. When completing group work, students will be able to rely on each other's strengths to get the work done, by allocating roles and responsibilities appropriately.

Through learning about strengths, students will begin to feel a sense of purposefulness that they may not have experienced before. They will be able to access and employ these strengths in your classroom (and elsewhere), and this will make for a safer classroom container, resulting in more serenity and less stress in your classroom. (In the next chapter you'll learn about your own strengths – little superpowers you can use to meet the world as your best self.)

How can mindfulness help in building a container?

As teachers, we can't control what happens outside our classroom, but we can work to create a predictable environment. We can co-create, teach, and uphold rules, procedures, and routines that will allow our students to not just survive the time they are with us, but hopefully to thrive.

We'll only be able to create and maintain this safe classroom container if we're present; if we're consistently paying attention to students and the dynamics of the classroom; and if we're honest about what's working and what's not. In a later

---

9. Lopez, S.J. & Louis, M.C. (2009) The principles of strengths-based education, *Journal of College and Character*, X(4)

chapter we'll discuss the idea of consistent reflective mindfulness practice in our teaching, but for now we're simply practicing paying attention without judgment.

Once you start to build the structure, framework, and opportunity for a safe classroom container, then you need to pay attention. This is your mindfulness practice in action. What is working for students and what's not? What is working for you and what's not?

It's clear that teaching is a bit like a dance. You just want to be an active participant in the dance, so you don't end up stepping on your partner's toes. The way to do that is to continue finding places in your day where you can bring mindful awareness; with that comes routine that students can count on. Creating (and maintaining) a safe classroom container is challenging work, so Part III of this book is all about how you can practice mindfulness more deliberately and keep filling your own cup while you aren't actively teaching.

Questions to ponder on the path

• What methods of creating a safe classroom container are you already employing, either consciously or unconsciously?

• What new strategies can you use? Establishing rules and procedures? Creating daily/weekly routines? Building relationships?

• How can mindfulness practice support you to create a safe container?

Step into action

• Decide on your primary focus in deliberately building a classroom container: rules, routines, or relationships?

• Choose one activity or procedure to do this week to start building this container.

• Support students to build their own relationships by exploring strengths, kindness, and/or mindful listening.

Featured five-minute practice: Listen For What Matters, aka Eavesdropping Practice

When you're in a meeting, when your students (or children) are talking to one another, or when your colleagues are chatting in the faculty room or at lunch, listen for what matters in their stories and conversations. You can do this even when you're not a part of the conversation. Listen with complete attention to their body language, tone, words, and other communication cues. Then choose to join the conversation or just use this as listening practice.

Supplemental resources

Check out www.teachingwell.life/pathbook for more resources to accompany this chapter.

Part III.
The teacher's life

Examine how the Path of the Mindful Teacher extends to all aspects of your life, because we want to reap these benefits in school and beyond

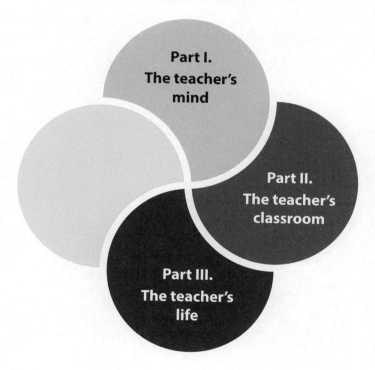

Part I.
The teacher's mind

Part II.
The teacher's classroom

Part III.
The teacher's life

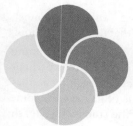

Chapter 6.
Learn your strengths

I now know myself to be a person of weakness and strength, liability and giftedness, darkness and light. I now know that to be whole means to reject none of it but to embrace all of it – Parker J. Palmer

Chapter objectives

You will be able to:

- Focus on your strengths rather than weaknesses.
- Determine how specific strengths can support your classroom teaching.
- Examine how your strengths can support your personal development.

Every summer of my teaching life, I excitedly marked on my paper calendar the days I had blocked out for planning my classes for the upcoming school year. When those days arrived, I eagerly analyzed the list of major and minor projects and assignments that I needed to cover, and the big pieces of content that were predetermined. I went through the process of printing out monthly calendars. I planned.

Hours would go by. Eventually I would look up, wondering where the time had gone. I was in a state of pure flow. I was utterly engaged in the process of planning my school year. I came to the blank calendar feeling not overwhelmed, but instead like it was a puzzle waiting to be solved. It was my nerdy, guilty pleasure. Those days when I worked on my calendars, arranged my room, put away supplies, made copies, created folders – those were sometimes the days that I enjoyed the most, even more than when the students showed up in my room on that first day of school.

Some of you may be nodding your heads in recognition. You may love planning too, and you may have all your materials neatly stored in a system that perhaps only you understand. But some of you may not love that part of teaching at all – you may create lesson plans only because you have to. None of us have the same strengths and weaknesses, and because of the diversity of the students we reach and the content areas we teach, this is a good thing. However, understanding that and *knowing* our strengths are two completely different things.

When I started studying positive psychology, I was required to take some strengths tests. What I learned through those tests changed how I saw myself. I learned it's not that I'm great at calendar planning, rather that my strength is in strategizing. I learned it's not that I'm a great keeper of items, rather that I have the strength of input (I'm a collector of ideas, thoughts, knowledge, *and* physical items). This knowledge opened up my mind and allowed me to consider my strengths and weaknesses in a new light.

What does this have to do with the Path of the Mindful Teacher?

After we've established a mindfulness practice and worked with our students to build a safe classroom container, we need to pave the way for us to continue these practices. It's much easier to continue on this mindful path when you really know yourself and what makes you tick.

As Parker J. Palmer states at the beginning of this chapter, to be whole is to accept and understand all parts of ourselves. We are who we are, and we all have gifts to bestow upon this world. The more we try to transform ourselves into something we're not called to be, the less we can light up the world with who we really are.

If you consistently wish you were the kind of person who likes to go to the gym, because you always hear how good it is for your health, but you really want to be socializing and taking dance classes, what will probably happen is that you won't go to the gym *and* you won't get to the dance class. If you learned about your strengths, perhaps you would be more open to activities and opportunities that put you in a state of flow in all areas of your life – work, play, relationships.

How often are we told to improve on our weaknesses? How often do we offer remediation to students in the hope that they'll perform better in a particular subject, while neglecting to emphasize the very subject or thing they are good at? It's not that we shouldn't acknowledge weaknesses and find methods of support.

But, generally, people feel a lot of pressure to improve their weaknesses to the point of mastery, and if they can't do that, they might give up trying.

Focusing on activities that activate strengths puts people in a state of flow. Mihaly Csikszentmihalyi,[10] the positive psychologist credited with popularizing the concept, told *Wired* magazine his definition of flow: "Being completely involved in an activity for its own sake. The ego falls away. Time flies. Every action, movement, and thought follows inevitably from the previous one, like playing jazz. Your whole being is involved, and you're using your skills to the utmost."[11]

When people are in flow, they're in a zone; their brains are active and efficient. They enjoy what they're doing, and it increases health and wellbeing. Although many of us know our strengths, we all may be guilty of feeling the pressure to focus mostly on improving our weaknesses. I'm not advocating only doing things that are easy and never trying anything new. However, by knowing your strengths and accessing them regularly, you may find a new way of looking at tasks. They may seem more enjoyable. You may realize why you love some things and start doing more of them. And when you do more of those things that activate your strengths, you will increase your wellbeing. It's one big, happy strength cycle!

Of course, we can't live in flow always, but we can design our time and our lives to maximize our ability to be in flow. In this chapter, we'll talk about our strengths; in the next chapter, we'll discuss finding mindful moments in our busy days. Once we've learned about our strengths, we can design our schedule, knowing those things that bring us joy.

A note on the dark side of our strengths

Just as teaching may have been a great choice for you at first, but perhaps it turned into a stressful job that sucked joy out of your life, unrestrained strengths can also be detrimental.

We can overcompensate for things that feel unbalanced by relying too much on our strengths. Let's take my strategic strength of lesson planning and curriculum writing as an example. The dark side of that strength is that if I get too caught up in planning, I become rigid in my teaching and never sway from the lesson plan. If I become so engrossed in planning that I never make the preparations needed to deliver the lesson well, I will not be effective in the classroom. I need to balance my love of planning with the reality of having students in front of me.

---

10. www.positivepsychology.com/mihaly-csikszentmihalyi-father-of-flow
11. Geirland, J. (1996) Go with the flow, *Wired*, www.wired.com/1996/09/czik

Similarly, if a teacher's strength is in performing, they may neglect to plan. They may spend most of their time interacting and building rapport with students, but not have a map of where they need to go with the class. It's important to consider what the dark sides of your strengths could be, and how those dark sides could manifest themselves in your classroom and your personal life.

Strengths tests to get you started

Because no test is perfect, a combination of strengths tests coupled with self-report will give you the most well-rounded insight. In my classroom, I ask students to take various assessments, creating a Strengths Record. I keep a copy and they keep a copy. Throughout the semester, we revisit how they're using their strengths to find success. We also try to learn each other's strengths, encouraging people to take responsibility for the activities that match their individual strong points.

VIA Survey of Character Strengths

The VIA Survey of Character Strengths is a free test with adult and child options. The premise is that everyone has a combination of 24 different character strengths (or things that they value). The test will help you uncover the ones you rely on the most and, by knowing these, you can more deliberately incorporate those strengths into your daily life. Look at your top five character strengths as a way to get started. *www.viacharacter.org*

CliftonStrengths

The CliftonStrengths assessment was created by Gallup and costs a fee, or you can buy a CliftonStrengths book and get a free test code. The assessment identifies talent themes, which can help you understand where you might excel and reveal the kinds of roles you might prefer in the workplace. The test may prove more revealing and helpful if you're looking for ways to bring some meaning to your job.

If you don't want to pay for the test, you could print out a list of the talent themes and highlight the five you most connect with. Investigate those themes and find ways to activate them in your day purposefully. See if you notice a shift in your overall wellbeing. *www.gallup.com/cliftonstrengths*

Me At My Best

Set a timer and write about (or draw) when you're at your best. After writing, summarize and analyze what you wrote, really trying to get to the heart of when you feel like your best self. How can you create more opportunities for you to be at your best? Try to make space for these opportunities in your schedule.

Reverse-engineer your strengths

In addition to identifying your strengths and thinking about how to leverage them in your classroom and personal life, I invite you to consider how to reverse-engineer your strengths to help you reach your goals.

There may be exciting ways that you can design your environment or classroom, or other shifts you can make, to help you more readily reach your goals. Think about a specific goal that's meaningful to you and relates to either your classroom or personal life. Now, try to figure out how you can use your strengths to bring you closer to that goal.

Remember, this stage on the Path of the Mindful Teacher is about building your teacher's life. You've learned the necessary mindfulness skills and extended them to your students. You've learned how to be still. You've observed your thoughts, feelings, and emotions, and acknowledged your scripts. You've worked to create a safe container for your students. But to maintain the serenity and calmness that you've found, you need to nurture and prioritize your whole self. That's why we start with our strengths.

Questions to ponder on the path

- How can focusing on your strengths rather than your weaknesses lead to a fuller life?

- What are the dark sides of your strengths? How can they affect your classroom and your personal life?

- How can you leverage your strengths to support a serene and calm classroom?

- How can you leverage your strengths to support your personal life?

Step into action

- Complete the strength test of your choice.

- Complete a strengths chart (available at www.teachingwell.life/pathbook) to consider the benefits and potential dark side of your strengths.

- Reverse-engineer your strengths by choosing a goal and mapping out how your strengths can get you there.

Featured five-minute practice: Obstacles as Opportunities

- Set your timer for five minutes.
- Settle in with a few deep breaths.

- When you're ready, think of a difficult situation or obstacle that you're currently dealing with.
- Really focus on what's making it an obstacle in your mind.
- Ask yourself how this obstacle could actually be an opportunity.
- Allow yourself time to really consider how this obstacle could present you with opportunities. Let your imagination run wild.
- Continue this exercise until the time is up.
- It may be helpful to journal about your insight after this practice, to help you solidify this shift in thinking.

Supplemental resources

Check out www.teachingwell.life/pathbook for more resources to accompany this chapter.

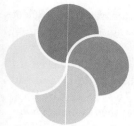

Chapter 7.
Find mindful moments in busy days

The way we do anything is the way we do everything – Martha Beck

Chapter objectives
You will be able to:

- Recognize that how you spend your time outside school can impact your classroom.
- Analyze how you spend your time currently.
- Design a plan to add mindful moments to your day.
- Set a goal to implement the mindful moment plan effectively.

I'll never forget when a janitor commented on my consistently leaving work on time at the end of the day. I was in my classroom later than usual and he was surprised to see me when he walked in. Innocently, he said something to the effect of, "Wow, you're never here past when you're allowed to leave. I always wondered: how do you get out of here so fast?"

I wasn't sure what to say. Only a few years before, right around year five of my teaching career, I had been on the brink of burnout and considering leaving the profession entirely. In the years since, I had dug my way out of many personal issues that resulted in a divorce, years of therapy, and, finally, a fresh start that I felt strong enough to take. Although I stumbled initially, in the second half of my first decade of teaching I felt like I had found a balance. I felt more secure in what I was doing and the choices I was making for my students. My grading was more efficient and my plans transferred more easily from year to year, because I was teaching many of the same courses.

In this particular year, one of my goals was to leave work on time, even if I had some items left on my list to finish later. I didn't yet have children and had no problem grading papers in the evening. My main priority was to leave on time, do something for me as a transition from work to home, and then complete a few nagging tasks on my teacher to-do list if I had the time and inclination.

I didn't pronounce these goals to anyone except myself. I was trying to do my job to the best of my ability when I was in school, and enjoy a different part of my whole self when I walked out the door. I hadn't even thought that anyone was paying attention until the janitor asked that question. As all these thoughts ran through my head, the only thing I could utter was an excuse: "I just move venues. I'm still working hard at home. Just need a change of scenery."

This one question triggered a cascade of worry about how many other people had noticed I left on time. Were people talking about me behind my back? Was I going to get in trouble? Did people think I wasn't doing my job properly? In retrospect, it's clear that moment could have thrust me back into the habits that almost caused the demise of my teaching career. The alternative was to pause and grab hold of what I'd learned through walking the Path of the Mindful Teacher.

Although it didn't feel natural when I first started on this path, I knew that if I wanted to continue teaching, I needed to provide myself with opportunities to practice mindfulness in all facets of my life. And that included setting clear boundaries, like leaving work when I intended to. Like pausing throughout the day to regain focus and clarity on the essentials. Like creating opportunities for reflection to see what was working and what wasn't. Like creating systems that allowed me to be more efficient while I was at school, so I could feel good about going home and turning off my teacher's brain.

Despite the doubting voice in my head, I knew I was a better teacher now than when I'd been working hard until all hours, dragging boxes of papers home to grade, and living in an unbalanced way. I knew that, despite the discomfort and doubt, if I wanted to be the best teacher for my students, I needed to be the best version of myself. For me, that meant developing myself as a whole human being, not just as a teacher. As Martha Beck reminds us in this chapter's opening quote, how we do anything is how we do everything. If I wanted to live a balanced life, I needed to bring balance to all areas of my life every day, not only on weekends, holiday breaks, or summer vacation. This is why finding mindful moments in busy days, the seventh step on the Path of the Mindful Teacher, is so important.

Why find mindful moments?

We find mindful moments in busy days to provide ourselves with a little respite, an opportunity to check-in, and/or time to reflect. In Chapter 2, we talked about the benefits of keeping a 14-day journal and I suggested ways to bring mindfulness to your free time, activities, and classroom. This chapter will provide you with some straightforward ways to bring mindfulness to your busy teaching days.

Teachers often tell me that they just don't have time to do these things. So, the first part of this chapter will ask you to observe (remember our classroom laboratory?) how you spend the limited time available in your classroom. Are there things you need to let go of? Are there areas where you could become less perfectionist? Are there places where you need to create healthier boundaries? Are there times when you need to leave work at school, so you can be present with your family at home?

It's no accident that this chapter follows the chapter on strengths. You now know the ways in which you may work best, or the kinds of activities you want to make time for in your days. You thought about your flow state and what you can do to activate that. Now that you have this information, you can make use of it as you examine how to find space for mindful moments.

Clearing out the stuff that no longer serves you and filling that time with practices and habits that *do* serve you is no easy task. But you'll find that small practices with incremental benefits will be far more effective than chasing a heavy, challenging, and demanding goal for months on end.

Before we can begin adding the good stuff, we need to get honest about how we're spending our time. Making a time inventory may be very eye-opening; at the very least, it will provide you with actual data about how you spend your time (remember to stay judgment-free as you do this). Then you'll need to decide what you want to do with the information.

I'll be honest with you. I wish I was the kind of person who listened to music to relax and unwind. I want to be the person who uses a soothing playlist as a transition between work and home, but the truth is that I love listening to political podcasts. Until I reach the point when this no longer serves me, I just have to find other places to bring more mindfulness into my days. Or, I need to view the podcast listening for what it is: an escape from my problems. If I see it and name it, I can perhaps figure out how it becomes more of a practice. Can I pare down what I listen to, choosing just a few of the best, most informative podcasts?

That's one example of accounting for time that means I don't have to change everything. We all have those guilty pleasures and the Path of the Mindful Teacher is not some form of asceticism. It's about taking an honest look at what is and what is no longer serving you – and then making a plan from that place.

In our world of increasing distractions, it's very easy to get overwhelmed by all the things there are to do and all the things you think you "should" be doing. Social media has given us a window into what our friends, family, acquaintances, and even people we've never met in "real life" are up to, and we think we should be doing the same. For all the conveniences the internet provides, it can be a nightmare timesucker that, if left unchecked, can lead us to feel inadequate, overwhelmed, and obligated to do more than before.

I'm certainly not going to tell you to find time by getting off social media and locking up your cell phone. Although, I will say that if your phone causes you stress and anxiety during the day, it may be adding to your stress in the classroom. Do you reach for it each time your students are doing something else?

So, back to the time inventory. You can find a "Where does my time go?" chart at www.teachingwell.life/pathbook. For a few days, just track the way you spend your time. It may be helpful to chart a few days during the week and then a typical weekend day. If there are pockets of time that you're using in specific ways, you'll get a fuller picture by including a weekend day.

Debunking the myth of 'no time'

Here's how I debunk the myth of "I have no time." We're all given the same 24 hours a day, and they are a gift to each of us. There are 1440 minutes in each day. We are in charge of how we spend that time. Now, before you go into analysis mode and get overwhelmed by all the tasks you tracked on your inventory, and all the things you need to do and are responsible for, please remember that *you* get to allocate this time. You are the one who needs to feel in the driver's seat. Try not to get bogged down by what you can't control and start thinking about what you can.

Look at your chart with fresh eyes. You have 1440 minutes – no more and no less. It's not that you don't have the time, it's *how* you spend the time. What are you doing that you love to do? What are you doing that you dislike doing? What are you doing that you have to do but don't like doing? What are you doing that you have to do and love doing?

Read through your chart a few times and see what comes up for you. Take a few deep breaths. You do a lot. I certainly don't want to take away the double-whammy busyness power punch that work and home life provide for us daily. So just be with the fact that you are doing a lot. There may not be children to take care of when you leave the school building, but you have many people relying on you while you're at work. There's only one of you. Sometimes it might feel that there's never enough of you to go around, but that's precisely why you must reclaim some of this time for yourself and spend it in the most beneficial way possible.

To get to the heart of what's essential, you may want to try a little mindfulness practice with the list of things you wrote down. Look at the list one last time and allow your eyes to close. Begin to take some deep breaths, inhaling and exhaling through your nose. It may help to breathe in for four counts, hold for seven, and breathe out through your mouth for eight. After settling in with your space and becoming aware of your breath, let the focus on your breathing subside and bring your attention to your time inventory.

You may want to hold the piece of paper, put your hand on the paper, or just leave it where it is. If you don't have anything written down, you may want to take a few moments to catalog the things you do on a typical day. Run through a montage of your significant daily moments with open-hearted awareness. If you're working with the tasks you wrote down, see if you can visualize this day from beginning to end. Run through each of these moments. Certain feelings may creep in, depending on the moment you're reflecting on. Just observe what arises for you, take a deep breath, and, when you're ready, move forward with your reflection.

Once you're done, if it feels comfortable, place your hand on your heart and continue focusing on your breath. The hand on your heart is intended to comfort you and acknowledge all the work you do. You are but one person, and you're doing so much. Take some time to value how much you bring to the world. How hard you're working. How much you care for so many people.

Sit with this for a few moments.

Now, I want you to bring to mind the most important things on your list. What do you *want* to spend your time doing? What do you *have* to spend your time doing? What do you no longer wish to spend your time doing? What is a waste of your time?

What do you want to hold on to and genuinely value spending time on? What do you want to let go of and it seems relatively easy? What do you want to let go of but it seems impossible? Breathe into how that feels. Is it impossible, or are you just struggling to see how this could be different? Who can you ask for help?

As you sort through these moments, begin to settle on how you want your day to look. How do you want your day to feel? What does your ideal day look and feel like? Take some time and just be with your ideal day. After you finish this exercise, it may help to journal some of your thoughts, reflections, and awarenesses.

The intention of this exercise is to show that we all have time and that how we choose to spend it is our individual choice. Do you feel like you control how you spend your time? Do you feel like others are spending it for you? Are there places where you feel like you're wasting your time or frittering it away?

Don't waste time beating yourself up or wishing that things were different. This book is about empowering you to choose serenity over stress and calm over chaos. A huge part of this is bringing awareness to your choices, so that your choices aren't choosing you. Remember the Four Noble Truths of Teaching: the way to achieve serenity and calm is to make teaching less about what we can't control and more about what we can. To thrive, we must be mindful of our responses to external factors and nurturing to our internal lives.

Make a commitment to yourself

Look again at your time inventory and make a commitment right now to try something different. The first step is to create a plan. Make a plan about what no longer serves you.

Here are a few things that others have committed to after completing the same exercise. See if any of these commitments resonate with you. You might want to commit to something different – the point is just to make some kind of commitment to start the process.

- I commit to starting my day without checking my phone.
- I commit to waiting to check email until after I get to school.
- I commit to leaving work at work.
- I commit to putting my phone away when I'm at the dinner table.
- I commit to eating sitting down instead of multitasking.
- I commit to taking a nap when I get home.
- I commit to single-tasking while my students are in my room.
- I commit to spending my lunchtime away from my desk.

As you can see, there are a few distinct places that often suck our time. There are probably one or two glaring areas where time disappears like a puff of smoke. Those are the places where you want to make these firm commitments with yourself. Remember that when you bring mindful awareness to these points in your day, you can make a conscious choice.

Instead of an absolute ban on certain behaviors, you may want to make an appointment with yourself. For example, make an appointment to check social media at a specific time for a certain length of time. Make an appointment to check your email just once after your kids go to sleep. Make an appointment to bring work home only two nights a week and not the other three. If you need to modify or change the appointment, treat it in the same way you would an appointment with a friend. This puts you back in the driver's seat.

What I've experienced in my own life – and other teachers have found this too – is that once I commit to just one of these practices, I start to gain awareness of other areas of my life. There's a snowball effect. Once you're looking at your day through a mindful lens and learning to be more deliberate, you'll begin to make changes – and they may start to seem more doable.

The myth of multitasking

Before we look at some tasking techniques that you may want to consider, it's time to debunk the idea that multitasking makes us more efficient. It doesn't. A teacher once told me that if she filmed her classroom during the day, people would ask what the heck she was doing, because she runs in so many different directions. Do you ever feel that way?

If you're a teacher, I can guess you probably do. We're pulled in a multitude of different directions. We're juggling a million different things. Logically, it seems like the best use of our time is to try to do a bunch of things at once. Well, it may sound logical, but science has shown us that our brains don't work in that way. For example, in a 2001 study, young adults were asked to switch between different tasks, including solving math problems or classifying geometric objects. The participants lost time when they had to move from one task to another, and they lost even more time as the tasks become more complex.[12]

It's far more efficient to focus on one thing at a time than to spread our attention over various tasks. When we extend our attention in multiple directions, nothing gets our complete focus. Multitasking is yet another area where mindfulness practice can help us in our daily lives. When we focus mindfully on one thing, we can more easily create flow, and when we enter that flow state, we can accomplish so much more with much less effort.

Time-saving techniques

There are many books, resources, and gurus that specialize in time-saving techniques. However, there are a few that I'll suggest as a starting point, because they've helped me to find more mindful moments in my busy days.

---

12. Rubinstein, J.S., Meyer, D.E., & Evans, J.E. (2001) Executive control of cognitive processes in task switching. *Journal of Experimental Psychology: Human Perception and Performance*, 27, 763-797

1. Stacking tasks

Stacking tasks involves grouping activities that you have to do frequently into bigger batches, allowing you to do them all at once. For teachers, I think of copying, grading, entering grades, creating lessons, and writing up reports/other paperwork. Can you head down to the copy machine just once during the week and make all the copies you need? Can you save your grading for certain days of the week, instead of grading each little bit that comes in? Or, if you need to grade each day, can you keep all the grading for one slot in your day?

When you stack tasks, your brain gets into a rhythm. It's possible to enter the flow state and you can become more efficient. Stacking may take a little more planning on the front end, but once you have a good routine in place, you'll be surprised at how much more quickly you can accomplish tasks. I also found that once I began stacking tasks, I figured out when the best times were to do different jobs and stack other things.

2. Pomodoro technique

The Pomodoro technique is built on the idea that we only have a finite amount of attention before we need to take a break. We are more efficient if we're laser-focused during a set period of time. The concept is similar to the brain breaks we give our students as they transition between lessons (see page 80).

The traditional Pomodoro technique involves 25-minute bursts of focused attention and then a short break, with a longer break after four successful Pomodoros. Because we often work with smaller chunks of time in our teaching days, it may help to assign one or two Pomodoros to our planning period and then take a short break before the next class comes in. If you're stacking tasks, you can use the Pomodoro technique to accomplish them.

3. Creating boundaries

Sometimes this is the hardest thing for teachers to do, but it's essential. If we practice mindfulness, we may begin to feel and see when we're spreading ourselves too thinly and need to set some boundaries with our time. We may also need to set boundaries with ourselves.

One boundary that I've set for myself is not overscheduling responsibilities after school. Because I've done this in the past and have experienced how I feel when I overschedule, I now realize it more quickly. I either change things if I can, reschedule, or make sure that I leave the following week generally free of additional responsibilities after work. It's a balancing and rebalancing act. When we're aware of our energy, body, and needs, it's easier to set those boundaries because we can feel the built-in gauge and our body's signals.

Remember that by saying no to certain things, you're saying yes to yourself and to other opportunities. Reframing the no may be helpful as you embark on boundary-setting. I highly recommend the book *Essentialism* by Greg McKeown.[13] It's changed my life and countless other people's lives. It taught me how to reclaim the time that I thought was out of my control. It's a great book to help you set healthy and guilt-free boundaries.

4. *Just leave it (but leave a list)*

We could stay at school every night and never go home, but still we would never feel like the work is done. The only time the work is done is when the summer vacation begins and you can finally close the door on the previous year. Yet, even then, we still need to dig our rooms out from the tornado that hit that year and begin preparing for the next school year. No, the work is never truly done.

I often give this suggestion when working with teachers: just leave it, but leave a list. Have a set time when you're going to leave work, rather than a set amount of work you need to complete. Leave yourself a list of the most important things you want to do the next day. That way, when you arrive at school, you already have a rundown of the things you need to accomplish or didn't get done the previous day. The list shouldn't include absolutely everything, just the most pressing tasks that need your attention.

Setting a hard time for you to leave work is essential because, again, there's always work to be done. You need to balance your time and energy into other things besides work. This allows you to choose serenity over stress and calm over chaos. Set a timer for when you're going to leave; when the timer goes off, write a list and go. You've been doing work all day.

I know there are times when staying late after school seems the only way out of the mountain of work. So, start by leaving (but leaving a list) at a set time once a week. Then see if you can add another day. And another. Find a routine that feels comfortable for you. You may find that you're able to adjust your expectations and get into the rhythm of leaving (but leaving a list).

If this technique seems impossible, take a moment to honestly ask yourself: who is putting the expectation on you to get these things done? Most likely, it's you who is imposing the deadlines.

---

13. McKeown, G. (2014) *Essentialism: the disciplined pursuit of less*, Virgin Books

Creating meaningful mindful moments

Now that you've brought awareness to how you're spending your time, and implemented some ways to be more efficient with your 1440 minutes, it's time to slip some mindful moments into your day. Remember that just as our classroom is a lab, our whole life is one grand experiment. If something doesn't work and you don't get the results you desire, go back and try something different. Mindful moments will give you the gift of checking in with yourself, and help you choose serenity over stress and calm over chaos.

If you'd like to try some guided mindfulness practices for creating each of these mindful moments, visit www.teachingwell.life/pathbook. Below are four places where you can add pockets of mindfulness, so your day contains some deliberate moments to regroup and recharge.

1. Quiet time

Take five minutes each morning to bring some focus and clarity to your day. This is a time to sit quietly, focusing on your breathing or the sounds around you; it's not a time for planning and making mental to-do lists. Take five minutes for quiet each morning and see how your days start to shift.

2. Intentions

Before your first class, write down your intention for the day and keep it somewhere you'll see it. Some examples of realistic intentions are:

- Carry less weight in my bag.
- Take a few moments and stretch before grading papers.
- Practice a few moments of mindful breathing at noon.
- Notice when my body tenses with stress during a potentially stressful meeting.

Here are some fill-in-the-blank intentions if you're stuck:

- I want _____ because I would like to be able to _____ .
- My intention is to _____ because _____.

Writing down an intention is a way to focus on a certain aspect of your day or behavior. Remember, it's more important to try out working with intentions than it is to do them perfectly. Write down the same daily intention if it's something you want to be fully committed to.

3. Reflection

Do a five-minute, judgment-free recap at the end of your day. End each recap by writing down one thing you're grateful for that day; however small it seems, write it down. If you'd prefer to do this exercise mentally, that can work too. Choose what you can commit to consistently and if it doesn't work, try something else.

4. Transition

Do something to transition between your workday and your personal time. This could be a five-minute quiet time exercise or a walk around the block. Whatever it is, commit to getting in the habit of making a firm distinction between your work life and your home life.

Please don't feel like you need to add all these mindful moments at once. Perhaps try one for a week, then a different one the following week. In a month, you'll have tried each of the mindful moments. Maybe you try all four each day for a week. See what you like and observe whether a routine is beginning to emerge.

If you want further support with adding these mindful moments, such as a daily journal sheet, you can download my free guide, *4 Simple Stress Solutions that Reduce Teacher Burnout and Increase Wellbeing and Self-Care*, at www.teachingwell.life/pathbook.

A note on habit formation

These mindful moments, coupled with the practices introduced in the CALM framework in Chapter 5 (see page 78), will help you to be present in your classroom and throughout your school day. They should be treated just like any other part of your daily routine. The more you practice them, the more you won't even have to think about doing them. They will become automatic.

Three of the best resources I've come across on the subject of habit formation are Charles Duhigg's *The Power of Habit*,[14] James Clear's *Atomic Habits*,[15] and Judson Brewer's work on addiction.[16] Another useful resource is Gretchen Rubin's Four Tendencies Quiz.[17] This may help determine how you respond to expectations and how to best support your habit type.

---

14. Duhigg, C. (2014) *The Power of Habit: why we do what we do and how to change*, Random House

15. Clear, J. (2018) *Atomic Habits: an easy and proven way to build good habits and break bad ones*, Random House

16. Brewer, J. (2016) A simple way to break a bad habit (video). TED, https://youtu.be/-moW9jvvMr4

17. quiz.gretchenrubin.com

Practicing mindful awareness will give you information about what is and what isn't working in the way you're spending your time, the way you're feeling, and the way you're behaving. From that place of knowing, you can choose to stay where you're at and get what you've always got. Or you can choose to do something different and get something different. The way to choose serenity over stress and calm over chaos is to be aware of our responses to external factors and nurturing to our internal lives.

You may be thinking that I sound like a broken record, but I keep repeating this idea because I want you to see that the choice really does lie with you. *You* are the one who chooses how to move forward from this place of knowing. It can be frustrating to learn that we are sometimes our problem, but it can be empowering to remember that we're also our solution. As we move into the final section of this chapter, I hope you can feel the empowering truth that you can do something different and feel something different in your classroom, and you don't have to wait for anything or anyone else to change. It's just you.

Creating a SMART goal

Now that we've discussed your use of time and explored how to bring mindful moments to your teaching days, it's time to make a commitment to yourself.

SMART goals[18] are a well-established template that has worked well for me, allowing me to hold myself accountable and plan for long-term, significant change. You may be familiar with them through work or a previous personal journey. We can't just wish ourselves into doing something different, but we can try our best to set ourselves up for success and anticipate any potential pitfalls. That's what this process of goal-setting is all about.

To make sure your SMART goals are clear and reachable, each one should be:

- **Specific** (simple, sensible, significant).
- **Measurable** (meaningful, motivating).
- **Achievable** (agreed, attainable).
- **Relevant** (reasonable, realistic and resourced, results-based).
- **Time-bound** (time-based, time-limited, time/cost-limited, timely, time-sensitive).[19]

---

18. The SMART criteria are commonly attributed to Peter Drucker's Management by Objectives concept, detailed in his 1954 book *The Practice of Management*. The first known use of the acronym SMART was in the November 1981 issue of *Management Review*, in a paper by George T. Doran.

19. www.mindtools.com/pages/article/smart-goals.htm

You could think about setting a SMART goal as you walk the Path of the Mindful Teacher. What is your SMART goal as you progress toward choosing serenity over stress? What is your SMART goal as you try to do something different so you can get something different? Are you ready to commit to your goal, so you can witness how it impacts all facets of your life?

Do you remember the janitor who asked how I always left school so promptly? Back in those days, I hadn't yet fleshed out my ideas on building mindful moments into my days. I just knew that I needed to create routines, frameworks, and strategies for myself and my day that were consistent, simple, and enjoyable. The janitor's question put me at a crossroads: I could either continue the work I was doing with my new schedule and routine, which had made me feel so much better, or I could go back to the tired, depleted, overworked, stressed-out teacher I had been before. There was only one possible choice. Even if I thought people were judging me for leaving school on time, I was determined to show through my actions that this path was better for me and, in turn, it would be better for my students.

I chose to double down on finding those mindful moments, and I know that my entire life is better because of it. I wish you the courage to find those consistent, simple, enjoyable moments. Commit to them – and to yourself.

Questions to ponder on the path

- How does the way you spend your personal time affect your classroom?
- How can mindful moments support your journey on the Path of the Mindful Teacher?
- What activities do you want to spend your time doing? What activities do you want to spend less of your time doing?
- Which mindful moments will you begin to integrate into your schedule?
- What is your goal as you implement this new plan?

Step into action

- Complete the time inventory. Remember, don't judge yourself – just chart what you find and analyze the results.
- Based on your analysis, make one or two commitments to yourself.
- Choose one of the mindful moments and integrate it into your weekly schedule.
- Create a SMART goal to support your commitments.

Featured five-minute practice: Rocking Chair Test

- Set your timer for five minutes.
- Invite your thoughts in without judgment: your to-do list, your expectations for yourself, etc.
- Then do the Rocking Chair Test. As each thought arises, pause and ask yourself: when you are past retirement, reflecting on your life in your rocking chair, what will really matter in the end?
- Focus on the things that really matter; try to let go of the things that don't matter as much.
- Continue this cycle until the time is up.

Supplemental resources

Check out www.teachingwell.life/pathbook for more resources to accompany this chapter.

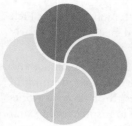

Chapter 8.
Discover the power of positivity

There are two wolves who are always fighting. One is darkness and despair.
The other is light and hope. Which wolf wins? The one you feed
– Native American proverb

Chapter objectives

You will be able to:

- Recognize that humans attach meaning (positive/negative/neutral) to situations.
- Describe the impact of cultivating positive emotions.
- Develop a plan for practicing positivity.

In my first years of teaching, I had a definite agenda for myself and my students. We needed to work hard, push ourselves, do more, read more. But doing more to do more was a vicious cycle that left me feeling depleted and may not have delivered real learning for my students. The pace at which we worked encouraged corner-cutting. Sure, they may have learned how to skim-read books and still get a decent grade, thanks to SparkNotes or the internet. But were they encouraged to dig more deeply into the topics, write for authentic audiences, or debate big ideas and issues that may have been a detour on our set route for the day? Not really.

If we did take a little time to go off-track, I felt guilty and scrambled to find a lesson I could scrap. I always compared my classes with those of other teachers who were teaching the same thing but clearly must be doing a better job. Honestly, I felt like a fraud. This constant hum of stress and anxiety followed me through my early teaching years, although I don't know if I even recognized it at the time.

In my undergraduate studies, I had been taught to assess through portfolios and reflections, and to conference with students to work through deep and meaningful revisions. I was encouraged to explore contemporary issues through great works of literature. I was shown how to use young adult literature to inspire readers and writers. But when I actually started working in a school, the honeymoon phase ended quickly. I never entirely lost the stars in my eyes, and I always believed that reading and writing could change a child's world, but my own pressure and expectations began to overshadow everything. After only five years of teaching, I was ready to call it quits. Clearly, I was feeding the wrong wolf.

After a particularly trying year of juggling classroom teaching and personal problems, I took the summer to recuperate and see if I could get a handle on what was going on with me. I sought outside help, found a support group, really took my wellbeing into my own hands, and generally tried to develop a healthier relationship with myself. In essence, I started feeding the other wolf just a little bit more.

When we discover our positivity, we can shift our entire perspective. As my perspective slowly started to change, I began to let go of my determination to reach a particular point and tried to focus instead on what we did accomplish. I gave myself permission to grade less but check-in more. I asked for student reflections and feedback. I tried new things and got curious about what worked and what didn't.

Over time and in small steps, I started to think about what kind of community we could build together. I tried to find ways to inspire students to *learn*, not just pass my class. I tried to encourage real conversations and communicate differences. I tried to provide authentic audiences to hear students' words. I used my strengths and mindfulness practices to figure out ways to connect with students and myself, creating an environment that celebrated rather than shamed them – and me.

The demands didn't change, but my approach did. I learned that not everything about teaching is a strength for me, so I tried to lean into where I *was* strong and help myself that way. I also found more balance throughout the school year, which translated into a more balanced teacher in front of the students. I was modeling balance for them without having to actually teach them about it directly. I was starting to embody the Path of the Mindful Teacher.

In this chapter, I want you to discover the incredible power of positivity too – the power of looking for those bright spots that you can control, instead of looking at all those things beyond you. If you know you're feeding that dark wolf, what's the worst that could happen if you gave the other wolf some attention too?

Each of us is wired for survival. Our brains are the same brains we had when we were running from saber-toothed cats to protect our lives; we're always scanning for potential threats. And although our situation today is distinctly different, our stress response remains the same. If stress hijacks our system because we equate it with a threat, then our amygdala is activated and cortisol is released more often, which leaves our body continually in a heightened stress response.

Mindfulness practice, in general, helps to realign our responses to stressful situations. Instead of reacting to those situations, we regulate and respond differently. But what if we were able to change our whole attitude and outlook on the conditions we encounter? If we could do that, then our entire system would begin to change: we would live in a state of neutrality, rather than one of enormous highs and defeating lows. What if we could encounter sun, snow, sleet, hail, rain, and navigate it all? We can. We will. That's what this chapter is all about.

Positivity is not Pollyannaish

First, it's important to debunk the myth that positivity is Pollyannaish. In fact, positivity is hard work. It's much easier to sit in a funk and settle into the idea that life is happening "to me" instead of "for me." By practicing mindful awareness and inspecting our lives as a scientist would, we may start to see where we slip into glass-half-empty habits and try to shift our thinking.

This is not to suggest that you should "grin and bear it" if you're experiencing an abusive situation or unhealthy working conditions. Not at all. Mindful awareness of your situation can help you tell a crummy day from an abusive rule or regulation. The positive here is that you're becoming aware of the unhealthy situation and can do what you need to do to take care of yourself. That is mindfulness in action.

Shifting from glass half-empty to glass half-full is hard work. But if we want to see things in a more positive light, we need to do something different. Positivity is not just something that seems like a good idea. It can actually effect real outcomes in our lives, as the positive psychology advocate Shawn Achor says:

> *"Your brain works significantly better at positive than at negative, neutral or stressed. Every single business and educational outcome improves when we start at positive rather than waiting for a future success ... productivity [improves] by 31%, you're 40% more likely to receive a promotion, nearly 10 times more engaged at work, live longer, get better grades, your symptoms are less acute, and much more."*[20]

20 Caprino, K. & Achor, S. (2013) How happiness directly impacts your success. *Forbes,* www.forbes.com/sites/kathycaprino/2013/06/06/how-happiness-directly-impacts-your-success

Life just happens

It's our perception of events that causes us to have either a stress response or a serene response. When we tracked our emotions at the beginning of the book, we talked about labelling them as unpleasant, pleasant, or neutral, instead of positive or negative. That was our first practice at removing the labels of "good" and "bad" from the things we experience.

Have you ever heard the parable of the Chinese farmer? It's a 2000-year-old story that's been passed down through the generations because of its timelessness. There are many versions of this story; the version that I tell here is reproduced with permission from the physician and spiritual coach Karen Wyatt.[21]

Once there was a Chinese farmer who worked his farm together with his son and their horse. When the horse ran off one day, neighbors came to say, "How unfortunate for you!"

The farmer replied, "Maybe yes, maybe no."

When the horse returned, followed by a herd of wild horses, the neighbors gathered around and exclaimed, "What good luck for you!"

The farmer stayed calm and replied, "Maybe yes, maybe no."

While trying to tame one of the wild horses, the farmer's son fell and broke his leg. He had to rest and couldn't help with the farm chores. "How sad for you!" the neighbors cried.

"Maybe yes, maybe no," said the farmer.

Shortly after that, a neighboring army threatened the farmer's village. All the young men in the village were drafted to fight the invaders. Many died. But the farmer's son had been left out of the fighting because of his broken leg. People said to the farmer, "What a good thing your son couldn't fight!"

"Maybe yes, maybe no," was all the farmer said.

Quite simply, we never know what life will bring us. Let's not get swept away in the ups and downs, and instead try to see the bumps and bruises as part of the journey. Reframing our situations positively is not necessarily about saying we're happy with them. We can see that there's more than one aspect of our reality. It's not all doom and gloom, and it's not all bright and sunny either. How would we know what darkness was unless we saw the light?

---

21. www.karenwyattmd.com

Positive emotions build resilience

If there's one thing teachers need, it's resilience. The meditation teacher Sharon Salzberg writes:

> "*Happiness at work depends on our ability to cope with the obstacles that come our way and to bounce back, learn from mistakes, make amends when necessary, and – most important of all – begin again without rumination or regret. This is perhaps the greatest lesson of meditation and mindfulness practice – that is what we mean by resilience. No matter what happens to us, we can learn to use challenges as opportunities to grow, increase our awareness, and learn methods for making future challenges more tolerable.*"[22]

The good news is that everyone has resilience. What varies is how well it's utilized and activated in the face of adversity. The even better news is that there are ways to increase our ability to be resilient. We teach our students about methods of building resilience – growth mindset, positive self-talk, positive thinking – but we may be neglecting our own need for greater resilience. Earlier in the book, we talked about stress being contagious, but our mindfulness, resilience, and positivity are also contagious to our students. It's important to acknowledge and understand how our behaviors can benefit others. We want our students to be resilient members of society; just as we model behaviors such as respect and diligence, we must also model resilience.

Our profession can be joyous, rewarding, and fulfilling in a way that many careers are not, but it also involves stress, adversity, and social and emotional exhaustion, for reasons that are beyond our control. As governments have cut funding, we've had to tolerate more than perhaps the average profession would endure. After years of stagnant wage growth, increased expectations with decreased resources, and the pressures of the Covid-19 pandemic, we are feeling the overwhelming impact, and our health and wellbeing are suffering. We build our resilience to fortify ourselves against the increasing demands of our work environment.

Building resiliency is *not* something we do to tolerate more stress and increased demands. Rather, greater resilience will allow us to bounce back from stressful situations and make a choice from a place of health and wellbeing, instead of a place where we feel stuck and victimized. Resilience is about being empowered in the face of adversity. And positive emotions build resilience because, when we routinely and habitually seek to find the silver lining, we can more automatically respond in that way during times of great difficulty. This is not to say that we don't

---

22. Salzberg, S. (2014) *Real Happiness at Work: meditations for accomplishment, achievement, and peace,* Workman Publishing, p.105

acknowledge feelings of loss or sadness as we move to positivity, but that we can see the full scope of the event and work through it in a way that empowers rather than destroys us.

How to practice positivity

There are many ways to practice being more positive. It starts with bringing mindful awareness to your present moment. Think back to your Mind/Body Connection Journal. Can you practice acknowledging when you feel a particular feeling, pausing, and being with this feeling? Just being with what is, instead of trying to change your feelings or responses.

Appreciate the awareness your mindfulness practice affords you. Greet the opportunity to practice adaptability. Welcome the exploration of your frustration. All these are part of the practice. They build resilience and help to rewire your brain for positivity. According to Salzberg, "When we're adaptable, we learn to focus our energy on areas of the job that we can manage and let go of the rest. When we take time to focus on the part of the environment we can control – most particularly ourselves – our working life becomes less emotionally precarious."[23] These practices will not only build resilience but they will also increase feelings of equanimity. This is similar to feeling calm in the center of the storm. Our classroom may be the storm at times, but our resilience will help us have equanimity and stillness throughout this rough weather.

Try building some of the following mindfulness practices into your daily routine; you may find that your outlook starts to shift. It will take less effort to find the silver lining and you'll become more resilient in the face of adversity – a great outcome for teachers who want to choose serenity over stress.

Heartfulness Practice

This is a practice you can do formally or informally throughout your day; it's a way to work with your feelings about people in a more positive, accepting way. You're essentially wishing positive things for yourself and for others, even people you don't always care for, and then extending this heartfulness to all beings, everywhere.

I encourage you to try this practice, even if you feel a little resistant. Sit in a quiet place and say the following phrases to yourself (visualize yourself as a small child if that feels more accessible):

---

23. Salzberg, S. (2014) *Real Happiness at Work: meditations for accomplishment, achievement, and peace*, Workman Publishing, p.114

- May I be happy.
- May I be healthy.
- May I know joy.
- May I know peace.
- May I live with ease.

Now think of someone you're close to and wish those wishes for them. Then move on to someone neutral: a mail carrier, a grocer, a neighbor you don't know well. Next, bring to mind a difficult person – not the *most* difficult person, but one for whom you have some problematic feelings – and wish those wishes for them. Finally, extend the wishes to a larger population and even to all beings, everywhere.

Rick Hanson's HEAL

Rick Hanson, Ph.D. is a psychologist and senior fellow of the Greater Good Science Center at the University of California, Berkeley. He explores the benefits of neuroplasticity and mindfulness in many of his books. In *Hardwiring Happiness*,[24] he presents the acronym HEAL to help you get a dose of positivity.

Have: to Hanson, this means having a great experience or revisiting a wonderful experience in your memory.

Enhance/enrich: keep the positive thought active in your mind. Enhance it by tuning into your bodily sensations or your five senses at that moment. Our minds often let go of positive thoughts and hang on to negative ones, so we need to work harder to make the positive ones stick.

Absorb: really let the positive experience sink in. This is a time to savor the experience.

Link: this is an optional step. After you've completed the HEA portion of the exercise, recall a negative experience that you might want to "rewire." Try not to pick something too hard. For example, I'll choose a student having an angry outburst in the middle of class. I have a generally good relationship with this student, so I recall what I really know about him through the HEA and then bring the difficult outburst to my mind. I also bring up a positive memory of him lighting up when telling me about a book he loved. I let the two memories mingle a bit. If I do this several times, I can create a positive memory association.

---

24. Hanson, R. (2016) *Hardwiring Happiness: the new brain science of contentment, calm, and confidence*, Harmony

Positivity practices

- **Practice gratitude:** write it down, say it aloud, share at the dinner table. Recognize what you're grateful every day.

- **One Minute For Good:** time yourself for one minute as you list all the positive things that have happened, or focus on one incident and visualize the positive aspects of the experience.

- **Write it down:** do a brain dump and just get all your feelings and thoughts down on paper. Try to get it all out honestly, and then try to let it go or embrace it, depending on what you're exploring.

- **Move a little more:** take time for movement that you enjoy. Whether it's gardening, walking, dancing, or an intense workout, explore what your body loves to do and try to incorporate more of that.

- **Have some fun:** schedule fun into your days, weeks, or months. Rediscover a hobby, game, or activity. Watch a movie that makes you laugh, go to a comedy club and laugh, or share funny jokes or memes with your friends. Fun activities can be simple.

- **Conscious kindness:** the best way to generate positive feelings is to do something nice for someone else. Deliberately holding a door or buying someone's coffee in line is a simple gesture that can have a ripple effect.

- **Cultivate connections:** send a note, a text, an email or even a handwritten letter to reinforce a relationship that's important to you. Make regular dates to see family and friends in order to nurture those relationships.

Final words on the power of positivity

Hanson says our brains are like Velcro for negative emotions and Teflon for positive ones. We need to practice discovering the positive, absorbing it, and re-evaluating to see how we can glean positive lessons from our experiences. For me to continue being a teacher, I had to change the way I perceived my job and how I understood my ultimate role for my students. I had a negative perception that unless my entire class got to a certain point, I was a failure. I needed to shift to a more positive perception, where doing my best to help students make progress was enough.

Practicing mindfulness makes you more aware of the way things are, but you may not like everything you become aware of. I certainly didn't like the realization that I would drive myself out of the teaching profession unless I changed how I ran my classroom. When these realizations happen, the key is to take those lessons and try to find a silver lining. This will help you build resilience in your classroom and in life.

Remember that life goes on. Our interaction with reality shapes how we feel on a day-to-day basis. The Path of the Mindful Teacher is a journey to empower you in your classroom and other areas of your life. Like all the steps, practicing positivity can be challenging, but I encourage you to commit. A consistent practice may alter your perspective, which can ultimately change your world.

Questions to ponder on the path

- How does the way we see the world affect our lives?
- What is the impact of cultivating positive emotions?
- What is my relationship with positivity in my personal/professional life?
- What is one thing I can do to practice positivity in the next 24 hours?

Step into action

- Practice gratitude (at the dinner table, in a journal, quietly on a walk).
- Pause for the positive (take a moment to pause and redirect your reaction to a certain situation, to see what happens if you "feed the other wolf.")
- Make a game out of these things. Don't take yourself too seriously. Have fun trying to find the silver lining.

Featured five-minute practice: Heartfulness Practice

- Set your timer for five minutes.
- Wish heartfulness to yourself: "May I enjoy wellbeing, happiness, and peace."
- Wish heartfulness to someone you love: "May you enjoy wellbeing, happiness, and peace."
- Wish heartfulness to someone with whom you have a neutral relationship (grocery store worker, postal worker, neighbor down the street): "May you enjoy wellbeing, happiness, and peace."
- Wish heartfulness to someone with whom you may have a difficult relationship (don't pick someone too difficult): "May you enjoy wellbeing, happiness, and peace."
- Wish heartfulness to the people in your community: "May we enjoy wellbeing, happiness, and peace."
- Wish heartfulness to all beings in our world: "May we all enjoy wellbeing, happiness, and peace."
- Continue this cycle until the time is up.

Supplemental resources

Check out www.teachingwell.life/pathbook for more resources to accompany this chapter.

Part IV.
The teacher's vision

Recognize your role in continuing this work in your classroom and perhaps beyond, into the wider world of education

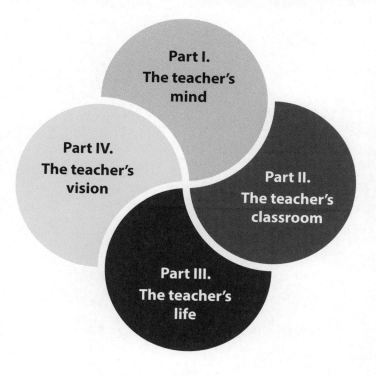

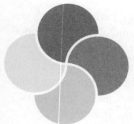

Chapter 9.
Reflect with self-compassion

You've been criticizing yourself for years, and it hasn't worked. Try approving of yourself and see what happens – Louise Hay

Chapter objectives
You will be able to:
- Recognize when your critical voice surfaces.
- Define self-compassion.
- Understand why reflective self-compassion is a useful tool in the classroom.
- Assemble a supportive community to walk this path.

I walked directly into the chaos. I was doing my mandatory hall duty between classes, standing at the door, greeting students as they came in. I had already interjected twice because of noise, directing students to sit in their seats and get out their books. I had already retrieved a lemonade bottle that was no longer in the hands of its owner, but had found its way under a desk on the other side of the room. As I walked back into the hallway for those final few moments, I didn't notice my heart rate escalating or my shoulders tensing. My body was trying to get my attention, but I wasn't paying attention.

The bell rang and I walked into the classroom ahead of my co-teacher, who is my saving grace. We can divide and conquer. We can give students more individual instruction and support as they navigate ninth-grade English. But even her presence didn't relax my tension. Feeling like I was stuck in a tornado, I tried to figure out why there was so much yelling, and how I could regain the control that had slipped away so rapidly in only the first 15 days of this new semester.

I don't remember what came out of my mouth, but a student's response set me off. I can't recall his exact words and I'm pretty sure I took them out of context, but I know what I felt like. I know I screamed for everyone to just get in their seats. I was shaking. Ready to walk out the door. Ready to not ever do this again.

My internal monologue sounded like this: "Wasn't it only yesterday that we talked about respect for everyone in the class? Wow, Danielle, way to lose your cool. That's all it takes to push your buttons? Your co-teacher is going to think you're a complete lunatic. I'm sure she doesn't yell at her students. Maybe she should be the teacher up here in charge. You suck."

If I could tell you that this incident took place years ago, around the time I began walking the Path of the Mindful Teacher, I would be thrilled. I could have followed up with all the ways I've grown and changed, and how I'm no longer so quick to react or listen to that critical voice in my head. But I'm going to be honest. This literally happened last week. Yes, just last week.

Remember the class that made me want to quit? This class has some similarities. Each student has individual needs and, collectively, there's a lot of personality in a classroom that isn't big enough to contain it all comfortably. But are these students going to drive me to quit? Not now, thanks to so many of the practices that are housed in this book (and, of course, my co-teacher!). The students were just being students, just like they were a decade ago and just like they will be five years from now.

But I've changed. Instead of continuing to hear that critical loop for the rest of the day, or feeling personally attacked by my students for not having any respect for me, I did something different. I recognized that the noise, outbursts, stress, and chaos in the room weren't about me necessarily. The students weren't doing this *to me*. Instead of feeling a sense of self-righteous indignation, I individually pulled different students aside for a check-in, came up with solutions during the class period to defuse the situation proactively, and tried to adhere to the class contract that we had just constructed together. This was significant growth and probably would never have happened if I hadn't been walking this path.

Why doesn't the critical voice just go away?

Developing our ability to reflect on ourselves and our teaching without self-judgment is one of the most significant gifts we can give ourselves. When we were preservice teachers, we all went through some form of student teaching; we had advisors who may have been brutally honest with us, and we probably had to be brutally honest with ourselves. It's almost certain that we were not great teachers when we started, at least in my case. I had to learn and make mistakes and grow. I had to be reflective – it was required. But it wasn't always a healthy or helpful form of reflection. I often berated myself about how I should have done something different or better. My inner voice told me I'd blown it because of something I did or didn't do, and that I had to do better at keeping my cool with individuals or groups of students.

It was intense, and it was a challenge to live in my brain. As I grew in the profession, I learned how to do better in certain situations, but the critical self-talk never truly took a hike. When I made a mistake or had a class that threw me for a loop, I resorted to internal insults and criticism that I would never bestow on my worst enemy. I always had thought that this critical voice was a guiding light for me: I thought it kept me focused on what I was no good at and what I needed to improve. But I know I would never want my children to talk to themselves like that.

Perhaps you also have an inner critic. Well, I'm here to tell you that this voice is not helping. Ironically, now that you're developing more awareness through mindfulness, you may hear this voice more frequently, at least for a while. The voice may seem to get louder as you become more aware. For it to fade away, it must be recognized.

Remember, the things we ignore and stuff away deep inside us will only manifest themselves in other ways. We need to acknowledge that this critical voice exists, and we certainly need to be reflective in our teaching practice. That reflective nature is essential to our growth as educators, but we need to add a practice to our repertoire to temper and balance our self-criticism. This practice is called self-compassion. As Louise Hay says, what might happen if you try approving of yourself?

What is self-compassion?

Self-compassion is the practice of treating yourself in the same way you would treat a close friend whom you love very much. It's seeing the humanity in everything we do, accepting ourselves for not being perfect, and acknowledging the hurt we feel when we hit a difficult situation. It's the practice of putting the bat down when we want to beat ourselves up with "should haves," "would haves," and "could haves."

Kristin Neff and Chris Germer are the leading thinkers in the field of mindful self-compassion. According to Neff,[25] self-compassion has three elements:

1. **Self-kindness vs self-judgment**. Instead of judging ourselves for all the things we do or don't do, self-compassion asks us to treat ourselves in the

---

25. www.self-compassion.org/the-three-elements-of-self-compassion-2

way we would a friend. We accept and act kindly towards ourselves when we fail, fall short, or otherwise don't live up to our self-imposed expectations.

2. **Common humanity vs isolation**. Imperfection is part of our shared humanity. None of us need to suffer in silence or believe that we're the only one who feels the way we do. We are all human.

3. **Mindfulness vs over-identification**. Self-compassion involves taking a balanced approach to our negative thinking. When we practice mindfulness, we can look at the complete picture and see situations for what they are, rather than inflating their severity or ignoring real problems. Mindfulness helps us to see our part in the situation and take responsibility accordingly, without overreaction or over-identifying with our thoughts and feelings.

When we practice self-compassion, we accept ourselves the way we are, instead of how we think we should be. Most of the time, we don't expect others to be perfect. But we often expect ourselves to live up to this self-imposed standard, and when we expect perfection, we are doomed to fail from the beginning. Self-compassion practice asks us to be gentler when we fail, because we will. To err is human.

We may worry that we'll open the door to slip-ups or let ourselves off the hook if we're too gentle with ourselves, but that's where the mindfulness part comes in. We bring mindfulness into our self-compassion practice, because mindfulness helps us see the situation as it truly is, rather than seeing it from the perspective of our critical voice or the voice of complete rationalization. When we bring mindful awareness to our self-compassion practice, we accept ourselves and our situations precisely as they are.

Take a self-compassion break

The idea of self-compassion breaks originated with Kristin Neff and is intended to be a quick mindfulness practice you can use when you hear that critical voice. The mindfulness teacher Melli O'Brien introduces her four-step self-compassion break on her website.[26] Thank you to Melli for allowing me to use the following excerpt.

> *"When you have a situation in your life that is challenging, painful, or causing you distress, take a pause for a moment. Tune into your body and see if you can locate, and feel into, where you feel the physical sensations of the emotion in your body.*
>
> *Step 1) is to bring mindful acceptance to what is happening. By doing this we can begin to let go of hardening against, and struggling with, what is*

---

26. www.mrsmindfulness.com/mindful-self-compassion

happening. So step one is to say to yourself either out loud or mentally: 'This is a moment of suffering.'

Step 2) is about realizing our common humanity and normalizing the experience of having difficult feelings (as we all do sometimes). There is no need for us to feel so alone in our experience or feel guilty or ashamed of what is a normal part of being human. In this step say to yourself either out loud or mentally: 'Suffering is a part of life. I am not alone in this.'

Step 3) Offering yourself compassion and soothing. This is a difficult moment so here we bring kindness into the midst of our pain. First, place your hands over your heart as a gesture of self-compassion, or if there is another gesture that feels right for you, do that instead. Then saying to yourself the third phrase: 'May I be kind to myself.'

Step 4) This is an optional extra step. Here you can also ask yourself, 'What do I need right now to express kindness to myself?' Are there words that you could speak to yourself like 'May I accept myself just as I am' or 'may I be patient' or 'may I slow down a little and breathe.'

Or is there anything you could do in your particular situation that could nourish you and comfort you? An action step such as: taking a warm bath, going for a walk in nature, meditating, calling a friend for support etc.

Through cultivating this kind of mindful self-compassion we can find connection and soothing when we're hurting instead of walling ourselves off or shutting down. We can be open to learning what our hardship may have to teach us (as many a wise person has said, suffering is often our greatest teacher), and we can allow [it] to humble us, deepen us and crack our hearts wide open."

What is reflective practice?

Reflective practice is the ability to look at our behaviors, interactions, and processes, especially in the classroom, and make a decision about how to move forward. It's the ability to describe, analyze, and then create action steps for classroom situations we want to repeat and those we don't want to repeat. The idea is to reflect on what's happening more objectively, not in a way that means you beat yourself up, but in a way that means you can see clearly where things went well and where things could be different.

You may do this reflective practice all the time without even knowing it, especially if you've been in the profession for a long time. You may adjust lessons, create new routines, alter seating arrangements, and generally make decisions on the fly because of what you were noticing or how you were feeling. Applying mindfulness will make these skills stronger. This is what I attempted to do on the fly with my students after I lost my temper. I took a quick self-compassion break, reflected, and then proceeded with some new strategies to try.

What is reflective self-compassion in the classroom?

Take some time at the end of the day, or throughout the day, to check-in with yourself about what's working and what's not. But there's no need to be self-critical when you're being reflective – in fact, it can be detrimental to your growth as a teacher. Reflective self-compassion means reflecting on your teaching in order to learn and grow and change, rather than beating yourself up for not doing things perfectly.

The idea is that you're doing your best on any given day. And if it's not your best, that will be revealed to you through honest appraisal of what happened in your room. When you combine honest appraisal with self-compassion, real growth and change begins. Combining these two elements also supports our Fourth Noble Truth of Teaching: to thrive, we must be mindful of our responses to external factors and nurturing to our internal lives.

So, what do we do with the realizations and discoveries that we make during our reflective practice? Well, we decide what is within our control and what's not. We can apply the wisdom of the Serenity Prayer to guide our choices:

Grant me the serenity to accept the things I cannot change,

courage to change the things I can,

and wisdom to know the difference.

When we engage in reflective self-compassion, we can divide the things that are frustrating or difficult into two buckets: those we can change and those we can't. Mindfulness practice gives us the wisdom to differentiate between the two. We recognize the things that we can't change, those things that are governed by external factors, and we let go of our attachments to those elements. We can only change the things that have to do with us, our internal responses, and our relationship to our experience.

Nothing may change at first, but *you* will. And because of the changes that take place in you, you will experience your classroom differently. It's such an empowering truth that you are both the problem and the solution.

The importance of building a community

It takes a special person to become – and stay – a teacher. This profession is not for the faint of heart. I distinctly remember making the conscious choice to become a teacher, and I knew when I made that choice that it was not for money or notoriety. I felt so strongly about giving back to kids what was given to me that there was no other professional choice I could make.

Self-compassion asks you to connect to the common humanity of your experiences. What better way to do that than to create or reconnect to a community of teachers, either in your school or beyond. You may already teach in teams or commiserate in the lunchroom about students, but what I'm suggesting is that you find a community of like-minded teachers who can lean on each other for support on this difficult road of teaching.

Because we work with students all day, it's essential to find colleagues who can be sources of positivity. A community of people who want to complain and point fingers wouldn't be helpful. Rather, it's essential to find people who want to make a difference and stop feeling victimized – people who want to live in the solution and successfully navigate this often-challenging work. I also advise against partnering up with others who don't understand the importance of mindful self-care, as this relationship may not be sustainable.

Get out there and find your tribe. Interact regularly. Perhaps work through the exercises in this book. Perhaps meet for a morning mindfulness practice. Perhaps share a walk after school before heading home. Find those people who can help you learn to be compassionate toward yourself – and you can be that person for them.

Questions to ponder on the path

- What does your critical voice sound like?
- When does your critical voice surface?
- How is reflective self-compassion a useful tool in the classroom?
- Where/when can you begin integrating reflective self-compassion practice?
- Who can be a part of your supportive community?

Step into action

- Regularly take mindful self-compassion breaks.
- Engage in regular reflective self-compassion practice.
- Find ways to connect with and create a supportive community, so you don't need to walk this path alone.

Featured five-minute practice: Mindful Self-Compassion

- Set your timer for five minutes.

- Think of a difficult situation that you've criticized yourself about.
- If you feel comfortable, place your hand on your heart (or give another comforting touch).
- As you bring this moment to your mind, say/ask the following to yourself:

  This is a difficult moment/situation.

  Everyone goes through things like this – I am not alone.

  May I be kind to myself in this moment.

  What do I need to express kindness to myself?

- Continue this cycle until the time is up. If appropriate, try to provide yourself with what you need as soon as you're able.

Supplemental resources

Check out www.teachingwell.life/pathbook for more resources to accompany this chapter.

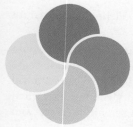

Chapter 10.
Continue along the path

Teaching holds a mirror to the soul. If I am willing to look in that mirror and not run from what I see, I have a chance to gain self-knowledge – and knowing myself is as crucial to good teaching as knowing my students and my subject
– Parker J. Palmer

Chapter objectives

You will be able to:

- Describe this path's cyclical nature and how this can impact the work moving forward.
- Evaluate which steps you'd like to focus on if/when you walk this path again.
- Determine what's next for you on the Path of the Mindful Teacher.

I still eat lunch at my desk almost every day, grading papers or finishing up a few emails. At least once a week, I stay at school later than I intended. More than I would care to admit, I react to a student's perceived misbehavior and then need to circle back when I realize that When you continue walking I took something personally. To put it another way, I've taken two steps forward and one step back on this path more times than I care to admit.

But I've also started listening to students more and building relationships with them as individuals. I take my job of mandating content a little less seriously and my role as facilitator of a classroom community a lot more seriously. I'm a little lighter than I was before as I progress down this path. I'm modeling my humanity in front of my students, in all of its messiness.

As I said to a colleague very recently, I can't imagine what my classroom would be like, or what I would feel like, if I didn't practice mindfulness and have these steps to walk. She laughed, but I was serious. Dead serious. The Path of the Mindful Teacher has been a way to get grounded among the uncertainty. A home base when I'm feeling unmoored. A choice when I want to move from serenity to stress and chaos to calm.

Hopefully, you've seen that the path never has to end. And, ironically, that's the last step. In this final step, you continue on your way, and if you're anything like me, it won't be once and done. When you continue walking, your circumstances, students, and school may be different than the first time around, but the steps will bring you back to mindful awareness. You may stumble or struggle on some steps more than others. Take your time, regroup, be honest, and remain curious.

Sometimes the path may widen as we invite others to join us on the journey; sometimes we will travel alone. Situations will change, but the path will always stay the same. Sometimes you may feel compelled to linger on one particular step, depending on what your mindful awareness practice reveals to you. For example, there have been times over the past 10 years when I've noticed an imbalance with my self-care and sleep. At the time, I paused and worked on Step 7: finding mindful moments in busy days.

After walking the steps initially, I found a lot of clarity by maintaining a consistent mindfulness practice (Step 2). Then I took some deliberate time to work with Steps 3, 4, and 5, exploring more deeply some of my scripts that I can now recognize as my implicit biases. Methodically bringing mindful awareness to my biases and addressing them was a profound step in creating a safer classroom container for my students. Without the Path of the Mindful Teacher, I don't know if I would have been able to address those scripts so fully. This path permitted me to be curious without judgment, something I might not have been able to do without Step 9: reflecting with self-compassion.

As Parker Palmer states in the quote that opens this final chapter, teaching holds a mirror to our soul. How we do things in the classroom is how we do everything. If we can see this journey as one of learning instead of shaming, we'll model for our students a lesson that we may never have taught directly, and we'll be more authentic teachers (and humans) than we've been before.

With this new-found knowledge in hand, it's really up to you how to proceed. The journey never stops – this path is cyclical. As you make your way to the next loop, you will have a different set of experiences to draw from, but the path will be marked with the same steps. It may be that just continuing to implement these techniques and bring mindful awareness to your classroom is the right path for you to follow right now. Or you may want to revisit certain steps and spend some time exploring a specific aspect of the path.

Remember, you never have to utter the word mindfulness to anyone, but your presence will be a present to all the people you interact with. As a result of these steps, you will more easily choose serenity over stress and calm over chaos. You will know how to determine your part in the stress you feel. This process will empower you to make different choices, focus on other things, and let go of what is no longer serving you, your wellbeing, or your students.

By following these steps, you now know how to be aware and present in your body during those times of stress. You know how to respond to those situations that push and pull you around. You've learned about your personal strengths and how to activate them. You've understood the power of positivity and reflective self-compassion. You can discern the situations that are yours to ponder and those that are simply not within your control. With these tools, steps, and exercises, you have a solid framework on which you can build your life in an empowering and present way. As a final review, let's revisit the critical components of these concepts, tools, and steps…

The Four Noble Truths of Teaching

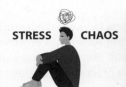

STRESS **CHAOS**

First Noble Truth
The teaching life is difficult, full of stress and demands on our time and attention.

Second Noble Truth
Much of our stress comes from not knowing how to manage the external factors, often beyond our control, that impact our classrooms.

Third Noble Truth
There is a way to lessen the stress and demands, and to live a more balanced teaching life.

Fourth Noble Truth
The way to achieve serenity and calm is to make teaching less about what we can't control and more about what we can. To thrive, we must be mindful of our responses to external factors and nurturing to our internal lives.

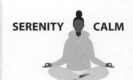

SERENITY **CALM**

Our journey began with an acceptance of the Four Noble Truths of Teaching. These Truths are the basis for walking the Path of the Mindful Teacher; they are what the journey is built upon.

The Path of the Mindful Teacher begins with realizing that the solution is in each of us. It always has been; it always will be. Now we need to do something different with the very stark realities we face in our classrooms each day, because we are the ones who can begin to solve our stress in the classroom.

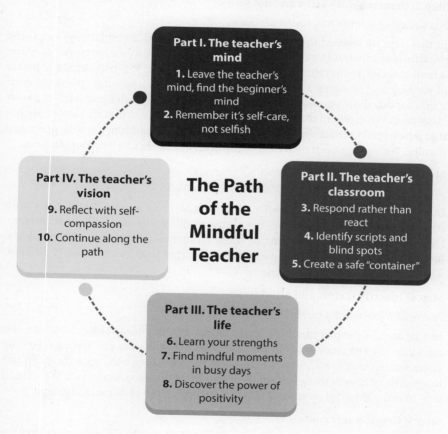

Part I. The teacher's mind
1. Leave the teacher's mind, find the beginner's mind
2. Remember it's self-care, not selfish

Part IV. The teacher's vision
9. Reflect with self-compassion
10. Continue along the path

The Path of the Mindful Teacher

Part II. The teacher's classroom
3. Respond rather than react
4. Identify scripts and blind spots
5. Create a safe "container"

Part III. The teacher's life
6. Learn your strengths
7. Find mindful moments in busy days
8. Discover the power of positivity

Step 1: Leave the teacher's mind, find the beginner's mind

Featured five-minute practice: Breath/Sound Awareness

In this step, we began by attempting to see our classroom, our students, and our routines with fresh eyes. We call that our "beginner's mind." When we take a step back and look at our world through beginner's eyes, what do we see? What do our students need? What do we need?

Step 2: Remember it's self-care, not selfish

Featured five-minute practice: Body Scan

In this step, we learned the basics of mindfulness practice and how we can bring mindfulness into our lives through everyday activities, a formal personal practice, school and classroom moments, and deliberate self-care. We discovered the power of pausing and bringing awareness to the things we do every day. We designated a spot for our daily practice at home and created space to anchor ourselves in our classroom. We explored the idea of self-care and recognized that it's not selfish, but that it helps us continue doing this challenging and demanding job with grace and dignity. We must put our own oxygen mask on before we can help our students.

Step 3: Respond rather than react

Featured five-minute practice: Working with Thoughts

In this step, we explored how to bring mindfulness to our interactions with students and to moments that are not always mindful. We explored our sensations, thoughts, feelings, and emotions in those moments before we react to students' behaviors. How can we learn how to respond rather than react? What is different when we choose a different response? Why?

Step 4: Identify scripts and blind spots

Featured five-minute practice: RAINN

In this step, we explored a little more deeply our often-ingrained reactions and emotions toward student behaviors, other school stressors, and feelings we hold about ourselves. We identified the thought patterns associated with the emotions to see if there is something behind the emotion that causes discomfort. We learned how to bring mindful awareness to our classroom scripts without judgment.

Step 5: Create a safe container

Featured five-minute practice: Listen For What Matters, aka Eavesdropping Practice

In this step, we considered how we can create a safe container for our students through the practices of routine-building, mindful listening, and mindful communication. We explored how to balance our focus inward when working with our own emotions, and outward when interacting with students.

Step 6: Learn your strengths

Featured five-minute practice: Obstacles as Opportunities

In this step, we considered our strengths and found ways to rely on and utilize them. We considered how our strengths can support us to overcome challenges and obstacles, and how we can use them to flourish both inside and outside the classroom. We learned to focus on cultivating our strengths instead of only on improving our weaknesses.

Step 7: Find mindful moments in busy days

Featured five-minute practice: Rocking Chair Test

In this step, we built on our increasing awareness of how we are showing up in our classroom. We took an inventory of how we spend our time, evaluating our use of this valuable resource. We explored some simple mindfulness techniques to employ throughout our days, specifically during our teaching times. We discovered some pockets of time that could be used for a mindfulness reset.

Step 8: Discover the power of positivity

Featured five-minute practice: Heartfulness Practice

In this step, we looked at the importance of cultivating positive emotions through gratitude and heartfulness practice. We uncovered simple ways to tap into the power of positivity and how this practice can transform our wellbeing from the inside out.

Step 9: Reflect with self-compassion

Featured five-minute practice: Mindful Self-Compassion

In this step, we discovered the power of reflective practice in our teaching and learned how mindful self-compassion can help us work with our new awareness. We explored the idea of letting go of perfectionism, accepting ourselves and our situations as they are. We chose to work with acceptance and non-judgment as we reflect on who we are in our classroom, with our colleagues, and within our schools.

Step 10. Continue along the path

Featured five-minute practice: Mountain Meditation

In this step, we acknowledge that this circular path continues as long as we keep moving forward. It may widen when different people accompany us. Continued walking on this path will allow us access to a potential solution to the stress and chaos for years to come. With these essential tools, you're equipped with the ability to handle the unknown challenges and ever-evolving dynamic that you'll inevitably face when working with children. By being grounded and practicing mindful awareness in all aspects of your life, you have the opportunity to be your best self inside and outside the classroom.

So what's next?

The next step would be remarkable enough if you just continued to practice mindfulness in your days. You would have enough to keep you busy, and the impact on the people you interact with would probably be quite profound. Therefore, I want to give you permission to stop right here and just embrace the 10 steps to the best of your ability.

However, you may feel inspired to pass on some of what you've learned to others. You may want to support them to gain mindful awareness, and that may be how you move forward. In order to avoid becoming overwhelmed, the best way to do this is to take an honest inventory of your strengths, assess your community's needs, and then determine your role based on that information. Opposite is a personal responsibility chart you can fill in to help you.

What's the plan?

	What are the needs?	What can I do based on my strengths and resources?	What is my vision?	What are the potential obstacles?
Personal				
Classroom				
School				
District				

Where can you start?

Take into consideration all the information compiled above.

Find a place where all these points align and write up a one- or two-page plan for how you can responsibly, meaningfully, and comfortably integrate mindfulness into your school or personal life. Don't forget to consider and address the obstacles or potential difficulties.

It may be that you continue practicing these steps in your own life and start to work with your children, friends, colleagues, and/or students, giving them some simple tools and perhaps sharing some resources. Don't feel like you need to give presentations or professional development workshops, or start a mindfulness group in your town. You're certainly welcome to do that, but it's not something you should expect of yourself.

As you continue walking this path, a lot of change may occur. You may already have found new awarenesses and a sense of equanimity, while becoming more grounded, resilient, serene, and calm in your classroom. The absolute opposite could also be true: your awareness may cause agitation and a desire for change on a deeper level. This could result in your wanting to do a different kind of work altogether. Teachers sometimes feel inspired to leave the classroom and use their gifts and talents in other ways.

Or perhaps you've realized that you want to do other educational advocacy work, focusing on the educational environment in which you work or your students' intense needs. That choice is beyond the scope of this book, but I've worked with people who have made that choice as a result of their awakenings on the Path of the Mindful Teacher.

The most important takeaway is that no matter what you do as you continue on this path, *you are your solution.* Keep the Serenity Prayer close to you and repeat the words like a mantra whenever you need them.

Grant me the serenity to accept the things I cannot change,

courage to change the things I can,

and wisdom to know the difference.

No matter our profession or relationship, if we focus on becoming our most aware self, we will be the best version of ourselves for our families, schools, and communities. We will be able to show up without becoming depleted and victimized. We will take on what we can and be present, without overextending ourselves and letting our wellbeing slip away. When our lives do become unbalanced, we will notice far sooner than we would have previously.

No matter what, consistent mindfulness practice using these steps will allow you to move through life more at ease with your needs. When your needs are met, you will be more able to give from a place of abundance rather than scarcity, and that is a win for everyone.

Some parting words

I wish you all the best as you continue on your path of becoming a more mindful teacher. It's my greatest hope that you've found this book empowering and feel more able to choose serenity over stress and calm over chaos.

I sat in your chair for many years and I still teach in a classroom every day. My goal, through this book, is to pass on the knowledge that has transformed my chaotic, stressful classroom into something that may not always *look* different but certainly *feels* different. On most days, I'm far more present and aware of what my students need and what I need, resulting in a different reality than the one I experienced day after day for many years. I'm better at creating boundaries that prioritize my health and wellbeing. I've learned to take things less personally. But I am the first to say that this is a journey that will never be completed.

Thank you for letting me share this path with you. The beauty is that it never has to end. Please stop to rest and pause when needed, and then continue if and when you feel so inclined. Above all, know that this path is always here, the steps are ever-present, and over time, hopefully, more and more of us will be walking this same path. Walk alone if you choose; create a community if that's what calls to you. With every step you take, you'll be able to embody this mindful awareness as you do the noble job of educating our world's children.

And please remember, the path never ends. You can simply begin again.

Questions to ponder on the path

- How is this path like a cycle?
- How does this impact the way you move through the steps?
- Based on your current situation, which steps would you like to focus on more intently? Why?
- What are your next steps on this path in your classroom, school, and/or community?

Step into action

- Create your personal responsibility plan (see page 137).
- Chart a plan of action for moving forward along this path.

Featured five-minute practice: Mountain Meditation

- Set your timer for five minutes.
- Imagine a mountain or picture one that you've visited.

- See yourself as that mountain: your head as the peak and your body as the base of the mountain.
- Picture the mountain as the seasons change from summer to fall, winter, and spring. With each season, the mountain is unwavering.
- See yourself as the mountain, moving through each season unwavering, solid, and balanced.
- Continue this cycle until the time is up.

Supplemental resources

Check out www.teachingwell.life/pathbook for more resources to accompany this chapter.

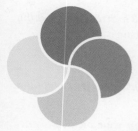

Further reading

Mindfulness in education

Erwin, J.C. (2004) *The Classroom of Choice: giving students what they need and getting what you want*, ASCD

Jennings, P.A. (2015) *Mindfulness for Teachers: simple skills for peace and productivity in the classroom*, W.W. Norton & Company

Jennings, P.A. (2018) *The Trauma-Sensitive Classroom: building resilience with compassionate teaching*, W.W. Norton & Company

Kessler, R. (2000) *The Soul of Education: helping students find connection, compassion, and character at school*, ASCD

Olson, K. (2014) *The Invisible Classroom: relationships, neuroscience and mindfulness in school*, W.W. Norton & Company

Rechtschaffen, D. (2014) *The Way of Mindful Education: cultivating well-being in teachers and students*, W.W. Norton & Company

Schoeberlin David, D. (2009) *Mindful Teaching and Teaching Mindfulness: a guide for anyone who teaches anything*, Wisdom Publications

Strengths

Niemiec, R.M. (2013) *Mindfulness and Character Strengths: a practical guide to flourishing*, Hogrefe Publishing

Niemiec, R.M. & McGrath, R.E. (2019) *The Power of Character Strengths: appreciate and ignite your positive personality*, VIA Institute on Character

Yeager, J.M., Fisher, S.W., & Shearon, D.N. (2011) *SMART Strengths: building character, resilience and relationships in youth*, Kravis/Whitson

Mindfulness

Brach, T. (2004) *Radical Acceptance: embracing your life with the heart of a buddha*, Bantam

Brach, T. (2016) *True Refuge: finding peace and freedom in your own awakened heart*, Bantam

Brach, T. (2020) *Radical Compassion: learning to love yourself and your world with the practice of RAIN*, Bantam

David, S. (2016) *Emotional Agility: get unstuck, embrace change, and thrive in work and life*, Avery

Harris, D. (2014) *10% Happier: how I tamed the voice in my head, reduced stress without losing my edge, and found self-help that actually works – a true story*, Yellow Kite

Kabat-Zinn, J. (2005) *Wherever You Go, There You Are: mindfulness meditation in everyday life*, Hachette

Kornfield, J. (2001) *After the Ecstasy, the Laundry: how the heart grows wise on the spiritual path*, Bantam

Williams, M., & Penman, D. (2012) *Mindfulness: a practical guide to finding peace in a frantic world*, Rodale Books

Building habits

Brewer, J. (2018) *The Craving Mind: from cigarettes to smartphones to love – why we get hooked and how we can break bad habits*, Yale University Press

Chatterjee, R. (2019) *Feel Better In 5: your daily plan to feel great for life*, Penguin

Clear, J. (2018) *Atomic Habits: an easy and proven way to build good habits and break bad ones*, Random House

Duhigg, C. (2014) *The Power of Habit: why we do what we do in life and business*, Random House

Fogg, BJ. (2019) *Tiny Habits: the small changes that change everything*, Houghton Mifflin Harcourt

Hyatt, M. (2019) *Free to Focus: a total productivity system to achieve more by doing less*, Baker Books

Levy, D.M. (2017) *Mindful Tech: how to bring balance to our digital lives*, Yale University Press

McKeown, G. (2014) *Essentialism: the disciplined pursuit of less*, Virgin Books

Newport, C. (2019) *Digital Minimalism: choosing a focused life in a noisy world*, Portfolio

Rubin, G. (2017) *The Four Tendencies: the indispensable personality profiles that reveal how to make your life better (and other people's lives better, too)*, Harmony

Turner, J.N. (2015) *The Fringe Hours: making time for you*, Revell

Positivity/happiness

Achor, S. (2010) *The Happiness Advantage: the seven principles of positive psychology that fuel success and performance at work*, Currency

Boorstein, S. (2008) *Happiness Is An Inside Job: practicing for a joyful life*, Ballantine Books

Hanson, R. (2016) *Hardwiring Happiness: the new brain science of contentment, calm, and confidence*, Harmony

Neff, K. (2015) *Self-Compassion: the proven power of being kind to yourself*, William Morrow

Ruiz, D.M. (1997) *The Four Agreements: a practical guide to personal freedom*, Amber-Allen Publishing

Salzberg, S. (2002) *Lovingkindness: the revolutionary art of happiness*, Shambhala

Salzberg, S. (2014) *Real Happiness at Work: meditations for accomplishment, achievement, and peace*, Workman Publishing

Selassie, S. (2020) *You Belong: a call for connection*, HarperOne

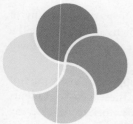

Acknowledgments

As a young girl, I dreamed of becoming an author but didn't know what to write about. From that ambitious girl to the writer with a semi-finished manuscript but no idea what to do with it, I kept the faith that one day the dream would be a reality. There are far too many people to thank, each of whom has helped me along this path. Know that I value and cherish the lessons I've learned from every one of you.

To Mark Combes at John Catt, for taking a chance on me and my little book idea. I thought you said yes to everyone and were just messing with me. But lo and behold, you were serious. The process was relatively painless and ultimately enjoyable, and you helped me reach the finish line with a smile on my face. Thank you for seeing in me what I could not see in myself.

To Isla McMillan, my editor at John Catt, for working with me during the final stages when I wasn't sure how the process worked. Your patience in helping to create the vision of what I wanted to book to look and feel like is so appreciated.

To Gale Morrison at John Catt, for helping to market the book and get it into the hands of as many people as possible. Thank you for working to help me find success through a process I had never experienced before.

To Jethro Jones, the first person to let me be a podcast guest and talk about mindfulness for educators. You've been an integral support through these past few years and I thank you for all you're doing for the future of education.

A big thank you to Nancy Lewis, a dear friend and former colleague. You were the first person I told about the book and the first teacher to read it; I knew you would give me honest revisions and tell me what you really thought. I was able to bring the book to completion confidently because of you.

To all the teachers and staff at Cocalico High School, especially all my colleagues (aka friends) in the English department. Your support and encouragement over the past 17 years has allowed me to be confident enough to pursue so many of these different endeavors. There have been many ups and downs as we navigate the changing landscape of education, but I wouldn't have been able to venture down this path without you.

To the administrators at Cocalico School District, for supporting every pursuit I've proposed, and allowing me to find ways to bring many of these ideas to students and staff at Cocalico. Thank you for trusting me to do this work to develop my ideas and methodologies.

A most important thank you to all the students I've worked with in my 20-year career. I was only 22 when I started teaching 18-year-olds, and I've been given ample opportunities to try, fail, and get back up again in the classroom. Each and every one of you has helped me learn a little bit more about myself. You know that I don't do it perfectly (not even close!), but I hope you see that I try to do better every day to be the teacher you all deserve.

To the teachers I've met over the years through Teaching Well, courses, and professional development, for providing inspiration that this path does indeed work. Your stories and creative implementation have been a source of the strength I've needed to continue this work. It's all worth it when we can support each other.

To my coaching partners, Kevin, Hope, and Kathy from Lewis University, for guiding and encouraging me throughout the publishing process, believing that this book would come to fruition when I was more than a little doubtful. You believed in me until I could believe in myself.

To Mrs. Nancy Sell, my high school creative writing teacher, who gave me a copy of *Long Quiet Highway* and encouraged me to write through all my emotions, thoughts, and feelings. You instilled in me the power of writing and the importance of a teacher who sees their students.

To Natalie Goldberg, for all the books on writing that I find inspiration in, give to others, lose myself in, and come back to again and again. With your guidance, I found the ability to keep coming back to my seat.

To Dr. Kim McCollum-Clark, for showing me what an English teacher has the power to be to her students. This spark was what kept me showing up day after day and year after year, in spite of the system not being what was promised.

To Sean Murphy, for showing my 24-year-old self how to write from the ground up, and then, 17 years later, editing the first draft of this book.

To Megan Cowan, Chris McKenna, Pam Dunn, Vinny Ferraro, and Christina Costello from Mindful Schools, for providing space to grow as an educator and as a meditator.

To Patricia Jennings, for being the voice I could finally hear in regard to mindfulness and education. *Mindfulness for Teachers* opened my eyes and heart to how I could apply mindfulness practice to the classroom.

To Deborah Mitchell, for being a consistent person on my journey as a teacher, person, and parent. Your support as a mentor and spiritual guide has been integral in helping me find my voice.

To Claire Stanley at Antioch University, for guiding me on my path as a personal mindfulness practitioner and encouraging me to write an everyday mindfulness guide for laypeople. Through your direction, this is what I came up with.

To Melissa Miles, for showing me the path of permaculture, and how nature can inform and provide regenerative solutions for so many of our world's problems, if we only pay attention. When we pay attention, solutions such as these become evident.

To Charles Eisenstein, for showing me a different way to view the world and its inherent potential. Your writings, thoughts, and philosophies are ones I return to when I get distracted or overwhelmed.

To Kelly Diels, for showing me how to own my voice, and let my voice and work lead.

To Heather Jo Flores, for showing me the transformative power and purpose of the heroine's journey, and the importance of exploring the intersection of permaculture, education, self-care, and writing.

To Kelli and Pat, thank you for being our family by choice. Your unwavering love and support have been integral in seeing this project through.

To Matt, my supportive little brother, and your family. Thank you for being the first official book purchaser. You've never stopped cheering for me and I thank you for that.

To my grandparents watching me from above, my namesake, Danny Nuhfer, and all the others who have kept watch over me as I stumble, fall, and get up again.

To my parents, for supporting me through all phases of growth (some more painful than others), encouraging me to blaze my own path, and instilling in me the importance of gaining knowledge and an education, because "no one can take that away from you, no matter what happens in life." Dad, you were also the first person I knew who meditated. I'm not sure if you were just resting your eyes, meditating, or a little of both, but that exposure lit a spark in me.

To Jordan, my supportive, loving husband (as well as beekeeper and stay-at-home dad), who cares for our young sons, dog, bunny, and our little urban homestead. You are my champion in all things. Your encouragement has enabled me to get up day after day and try to channel all these life experiences into something that can be of benefit to others. Our journey will forever continue.

And, finally, to my boys. You are the reason I've put myself out there and tried to do hard things. I can now tell you that with a lot of hard work and a little luck, dreams can (and do) come true.

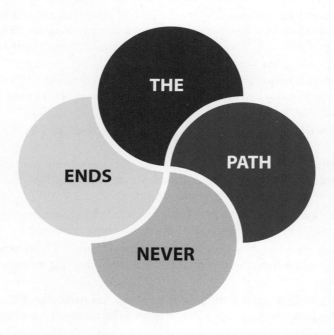